SOAP MAKING FOR BEGINNERS

Learn How to Make a Fragrant and Colorful Soap at Home

(Step-by-step Guide for Diy Soaps to Start Up a Business)

Sherri Davis

Published by Oliver Leish

Sherri Davis

All Rights Reserved

Soap Making for Beginners: Learn How to Make a Fragrant and Colorful Soap at Home (Step-by-step Guide for Diy Soaps to Start Up a Business)

ISBN 978-1-77485-077-0

All rights reserved. No part of this guide may be reproduced in any form without permission in writing from the publisher except in the case of brief quotations embodied in critical articles or reviews.

Legal & Disclaimer

The information contained in this book is not designed to replace or take the place of any form of medicine or professional medical advice. The information in this book has been provided for educational and entertainment purposes only.

The information contained in this book has been compiled from sources deemed reliable, and it is accurate to the best of the Author's knowledge; however, the Author cannot guarantee its accuracy and validity and cannot be held liable for any errors or omissions. Changes are periodically made to this book. You must consult your doctor or get professional medical advice before using any of the suggested remedies, techniques, or information in this book.

Upon using the information contained in this book, you agree to hold harmless the Author from and against any damages, costs, and expenses, including any legal fees potentially resulting from the application of any of the information provided by this guide. This disclaimer applies to any damages or injury caused by the use and application, whether directly or indirectly, of any advice or information presented, whether for breach of contract, tort, negligence, personal injury, criminal intent, or under any other cause of action.

You agree to accept all risks of using the information presented inside this book. You need to consult a professional medical practitioner in order to ensure you are both able and healthy enough to participate in this program.

Table of Contents

INTRODUCTION 1

CHAPTER 1: SOAP MAKING INGREDIENTS 3

CHAPTER 2: THE HISTORY OF SOAP 11

CHAPTER 3: HOT PROCESS AND COLD PROCESS SOAP MAKING 17

CHAPTER 4: SOAP MAKING 101 26

CHAPTER 5: UNDERSTANDING THE BASICS 43

CHAPTER 6: 3 SOAP MAKING TECHNIQUES 47

CHAPTER 7: SOAP MAKING FOR BOREDOM 68

CHAPTER 8: SAFETY PROCEDURES: WORKING WITH ALKALI 75

CHAPTER 9: WHAT IS SOAP MADE FROM? 96

CHAPTER 10: WHY SHOULD YOU MAKE YOUR OWN SOAP? 102

CHAPTER 11: WHY YOU SHOULD TOSS YOUR COMMERCIALLY-PRODUCED SOAPS 116

CHAPTER 12: SOAP MAKING MYTHS DEBUNKED 131

CHAPTER 13: SOAP MAKING INGREDIENTS YOU WILL NEED 136

CHAPTER 14: OTHER PRODUCTS TO MAKE AT HOME 154

    4.1 MARSEILLE SOAP 157

    4.3 VANILLA SOAP 163

CHAPTER 15: BEST HOMEMADE SOAP RECIPES 167

CONCLUSION 179

Introduction

The book contains content that will help you make a sweet-smelling soap, that is up to your standards. Since most people don't like what they are currently using.

It is common to find out that most people are repulsed by strong scented soaps, they get allergies and cannot stop sneezing or coughing due to the strong scents. Many fragrances used in the soaps might not be what you want or the color and shape do not appeal to you at all. For others, the soaps they are using are harsh on their skins, trying to find the right soap for your skin and to your preference is a tad difficult.

To help you with this, learn to make your own soap from the comfort of your house. Make the soap with the right essential oils that are beneficial to your skin long-term and get it to have the right scent and be in the shape and color you want.

The book contains recipes that can be used to create soaps for your family, pets, loved ones with sensitive skins and for your own muse.

In detail, the content here will help you learn some mistakes to avoid when making the soap as they are bound to happen and what you can do to avoid such.

The book has a plethora of information that will guide you through this process, you surely don't want to miss out. Open it up and enjoy :)

Chapter 1: Soap Making Ingredients

There are many different soap making ingredients that can be used to create soap at home. Whether it's a base, fat, oil, nutrient, natural preservative essential oil or colorant each substance has specific benefits for soap making, and will add unique characteristics to your finished product.

Before you use any ingredient for all natural soap it's essential that you know exactly what it is and what it will do to your finished product. In fact, that's the purpose of this page!

Are you looking to learn only about one specific ingredient? That's not a problem either! Just scroll down to the list of ingredients and click on the one you want to learn more about. If you don't see what you're looking for, contact me and I will be more then happy to write a page telling you everything I know about that particular ingredient.

Keep in mind that the right ingredients for soap must be added for saponification to occur. In this chemical reaction, an acid reacts with a base to form a salt. The salt is actually your soap!

What ingredient for all natural soap do I use as a base? Personally, I use a substance called lye for soap making (also known as sodium hydroxide). Although most soap makers swear by this particular base, you can also use potash (potassium hydroxide).

Lye tends to produce a better and harder bar of soap whereas potash produces a not so nice softer bar of soap. To be honest with you, I would only consider using potash for a base when making liquid soaps.

Choosing your base doesn't exactly allow you to explore your creativity. One of the fun parts about soap making, however, is that you can create many different types of soap by varying the acid that reacts with the base. This variant in your soap recipe causes your creation to take on its own unique form.

Here's a list of the acids that you can use to make soap:

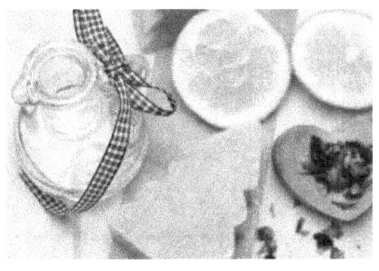

Avocado Oil for Soap Making:

Using avocado oil for soap making will increase the conditioning properties of your finished product and add creaminess to the soap's lather. Avocado oil also has wonderful skin care advantages such as a high content of vitamin A, D and E.

Coconut Oil for Soap Making

Many soap makers use coconut oil for soap making because of the incredible lather it produces, the hardness it adds to the soap, and, when used in moderation, its great moisturizing abilities.

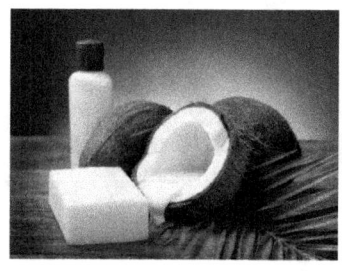

Castor Oil for Soap Making:

Pretty much all soap makers who use castor oil for soap making swear by its effectiveness for adding an amazing lather and great moisturizing properties to the finished product.

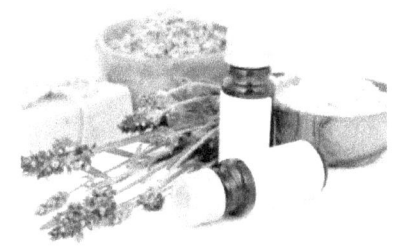

Cottonseed Oil:

Although some soap makers use cottonseed oil to make soap, I recommend that you do not. Unfortunately, there are several negatives that cause this oil to be unappealing for soap making. We will talk about those negatives below.

Olive Oil Soap Making:

On this page, we are going to learn about olive oil soap making and some key tips for creating a successful batch. Making olive oil soap is a ton of fun and the product that this oil produces is wonderful for the skin!

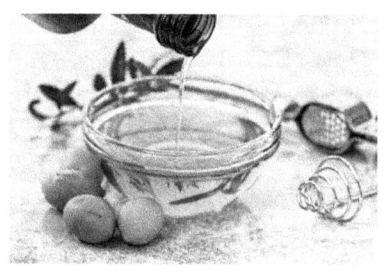

Shea Butter for Soap Making:

Using shea butter for soap making will add a wonderful creamy lather, great conditioning properties and some hardness to your soap.

Tallow Soap Making:

Instead of sticking with all vegetable oils, some soap makers use beef tallow for soap making. Admitantly, I am not an expert in tallow soap making. In fact, at the time of this writing, I have never made tallow soap as I try to keep my creations 100% animal product free. Despite the negative stigma within the vegetarian and vegan communities (and even some other communities), there are some benefits of using tallow for soap making.

Lard Soap Making

Many love using lard for soap making to add a creamy lather, conditioning properties and some hardness to the finished product. Although it does add beneficial properties to your soap, you need to be aware that it is not great for your label appeal. In fact, some people will avoid your products all together if they see that you use lard, or any other animal fat! On the other side of the spectrum, some consumers and soap makers love lard soap and will use and make nothing else!

Kukui Nut Oil for Soap Making

When using kukui nut oil for soap making you will add a stable lather, great conditioning properties and an often reported silky feel to your finished product.

Let's take a look at the fatty acid, iodine and SAP values for this oil:

Chapter 2: The History Of Soap

While people of ancient cultures, bathed infrequently on rivers or lakes. The earliest recorded production of soap-like materials dates back to 2800 BC in ancient Babylon.A soap formula consisting of water, alkali, and cassia oil.

TheEbers papyrusindicates that the ancient Egyptians bathed regularly and combined animal and vegetable oils with alkaline salts to create soap. It is also known that from Egyptian documents that a soap-like substance was used in the preparation of wool for weaving.

In the reign ofNabonidus it is said that a recipe for soap consisted of ashes, cypress oil and seed were made.

In Ancient Roman era a popular Legend claims soap takes its name from a supposed Mount Sapo, where animal sacrifices were supposed to have taken place. By ashes from fires with sacrifices and with water to produce soap, but there is no evidence of a Mount Sapo in the Roman. The Latinwordsaposimply means soap. It was likely borrowed from an early Germanic language.

Apart from that Zosimos of Panopolis, describes soap and soapmaking using lye and prescribes washing to carry away impurities from the body and clothes.

In Ancient China a similar to soap was manufactured from the seeds ofGleditsia sinensis. A mixture of pig pancreas and plant ash called Zhu yi zi.

In Middle East as a 12th-century Islamic document describes the process of soap making.It mentions the key ingredient,alkali, which later become crucial to modern chemistry, originating fromashes.

By the 13th century, the manufacture of soap industrialized in the Islamic world.

In Medieval Europe soap-making was well known in Italy and Spain.TheCarolingiancapitularyDe Villis dating to around 800, representing the royal will ofCharlemagne, mentions soap as being one of the products the royal estates are to tally.

Soapmaking began in theKingdom of Englandabout 1200 and it is mentioned as women's work.

In France, by the second half of the 15th century, the semi-industrialized professional manufacture of soap was concentrated and supplied France.

Better soaps were later produced in Europe from the 16th century, using vegetable oils such asolive oil as opposed to animal fats. Many of these soaps are still produced, both industrially and by small artisans.

In modern times, the use of soap has become in commonplace. Industrially manufactured bar soaps first became available in the late 18th century, as advertising campaigns in Europe and America promoted popular awareness of the relationship between health and cleanliness.

Until theIndustrial Revolution, soaps were produced on a small scale and were rough. In 1780James Keirestablished a chemical work, for the manufacture of alkali from the sulfates ofpotashand soda, to which he afterwards added a soap manufactory. Later on Andrew Pears started making a high-quality, transparent soap in 1807inLondon.

In the 1850s William Gossageproduced a low-priced, good-quality soap .Robert Spear Hudsonbegan manufacturing a soap powder in 1837, initially by grinding the soap with amortar and pestle.

In 1865, William Shepphard patented a liquid version of soap, and in 1898, B.J. Johnson developed a soap made of palm and olive oils. He made his company and Palmolive brand soap that same year. This new brand of the new kind of soap became popular rapidly, and to such a degree that B.J. Johnson Soap Company changed its name to Palmolive.

In the early 1900s, other companies began to develop their own liquid soaps. Such products as Tide and Pine-Sol appeared on the market.

Today, bar soap is made in a three-step process. First, oils and fats are combined with alkali to produce a mixture of neat soap, water and glycerol in a method called saponification. Next, the mixture is dried to greatly reduce its water content. Lastly, the dried, plain soap is mixed with fragrance, color and other additives, and then extruded into bars.

Modern soap is not limited to bars, however, with liquid soap and hand sanitizer quickly overtaking the market. In fact, in 2011 Americans spent more on liquid soap than bar soap. So this begs the question, which soap should I use? The answer is harder to find than you might think.

Chapter 3: Hot Process And Cold Process Soap Making

We already know that there's a difference between the hot process and the cold process. In the cold process, you just mix your oils with your lye water, pour into the mold, and let it do its thing, leave it for 24 hours, and it'll saponify on its own. In the hot process, you measure oils in your lye; you cook it, you're forcing that saponification to occur. So, basically, that's what it is about.

Main differences

The number one thing is appearance. In the hot process, the surfaces usually come out rugged, and it's not as creamy-looking as a cold process bar would look. So number one is the difference in appearance. There are soap makers that have gotten this craft honed to where they can always make it look better. There are different tricks to do that; I know that they add yogurt, sodium lactate, extra water. it is just different things you can do to make the surface look better.

The second thing has to do with how you use it; you can use hot process immediately like right when it's in the crockpot when it cools down, you can mold it together and use it. Aside from the actual physical temperature of the soap, it's perfectly safe to use, it has been saponified, and it is fine.

Labeling and Wrapping Of Your Soaps

Go to the grocery store and get an inexpensive clear plastic food wrap (this is the first equipment). Ensuring that your mountain for soap is wrapped in a professional and attractive manner requires a heat gun. You can find this in the hardware store in the paint section, or you can use a rubber-stamping embossing gun, but no hairdryers, they don't get warm enough.

STEP 1

The first step to making a professional-looking wrapped bar of soap is to tear off a piece of the clear plastic wrap, pull the ends tight over the bar of soap, cut off any extra you have; this will create an unsightly bulge if you do not do it like that. As the heat gun is low, heat the back of the wrap, you'll notice the plastic search shrinking up. Once it shrunk up, turn this over. Now, heat the sides of the soap to the other; this is important. Then gently hit the top of the soap with a little bit of heat. You can apply a label to the back of it to finish the entire thing off. This method also works for round ovals or even slightly strong bars. So, the first steps, pull a piece of your clear plastic wrap off. Pull the size of the plastic wrap up and over the soap, hit the back of the soap with heat. Once it's fully heated, turn this over to the sides and the top. Put a finishing label on it.

Or

Pull up the case of your clear plastic wrap off. Pull it gently over the entire bar soap. Cut the excess off, hit the back of the soap with some heat, hit the side of the soap with heat, and then do the top, very gently; if you don't do the top gently enough, you can melt your bar. So, the key to using your heat gun is short bursts of heat, or else your professionally wrapped bar soap may turn into a puddle of soap.

STEP 2

Now let's talk about other ways to package yourself; you can use soap boxes. Brambleberry.com carries two different kinds of soapboxes: the brown soapbox and the other is the white soapbox. The brown soapbox comes assembled in two pieces, the actual box and then the sleeve that goes over it. To make the box, first, fold all the pieces of the pre-scored box. This will make it easier to fold, then take the short sides and flip them up. Take the long sides and track the short sides. Finally, using the tags, push down firmly on the entire thing. Put your soap into the box, and the entire thing stays together. Take your sleeve. Push it gently over the box. Wrap this with a little bit of ribbon, put a label on it, and you're done.

The white box also comes flat in shipping. This is a little bit easier to put together, all you need to do is pop out all the edges, and you're done. Flip your bars open, put a ribbon around it, and put a label on the professionally packaged bar of soap. However, the soap is still in a box, but that doesn't mean that the box is airtight and will keep the air away from the soap. So the soap might even sweat, or just dry up and become an unsightly massive.

STEP 3

Some other options for wrapping your soap is the organza bags. They come in all kinds of shapes, colors, and sizes. They are used to make wedding gifts. Make sure you have wrapped your soap first with the clear plastic wrap and then wrap your soap with a wrapping paper and a little bit of ribbon, put a nice label on it, and its beautifully wrapped up.

Promoting Your Business

1. Figure out a target audience

So the first thing you need to do is figure out the type of population you want to sell to; for example, if you want to sell to middle-aged women, you should focus on marketing your products that have anti-aging properties. If you want to market to young adults, try to focus on the products that have skin brightening dark circles eliminating properties, so once you know what type of audience you want to sell to, then you move to the second step.

2. Choose your platform

You need to choose your marketing platform; you can either choose from Facebook ads, Instagram, or even contact some influencers so they can promote your product in their pages, and maybe even talk to storefronts so that they can put your products in display. The most important thing about this is that you think outside the box.

3. Collaborate with others

Try contacting stores to add your soap in the booth stand in malls, try contacting restaurants, bigger brands that you might be surprised that they will be, they will be willing to sell your products. Try operating with a bigger brand. They might or might not pay you for your products, but you will get a lot of exposure; some of the brands that might be good ideas are the ones who do monthly bar subscriptions, you can try contacting them.

5. Participating in local craft fairs

Try participating in local craft fairs; you might not sell a lot as you might think you will but keep in mind that word of mouth goes a long way

6. A brand that catches the attention

If you will do online marketing, your branding needs to be on point, by branding I mean your logo, the way you package your soap, the way you present them, it needs to catch people's attention, also try contacting big YouTubers in your area, make videos with them

7. Give out samples to locals

You should give out samples to the locals around you. Many people like free stuff, and not everyone is up to buying $10 soap if they're not sure they're going to like it. Try giving out samples; you can also sell those samples for $1-$2 depending on how big you make them; like I said, word of mouth goes a long way. You can also try contacting bloggers in your local area. If you have any, try collaborating with them, making videos with them. And some of them might say yes. Others might be too shy to approach other people that way. But you don't lose anything by asking, or sending emails or making calls to put yourself out there.

Chapter 4: Soap Making 101

Fundamentally, soap making involves mixing animal or vegetable fats that has a strong alkaline, usually a lye.

This process, also known as "saponification", is the chemical reaction between the mentioned elements.

For a beginner, it is highly suggested that the "melt and pour" method is the easiest process to start making soap. For instance, to execute this process, all you are required to do is melt down a premade soap base on a stove or in your microwave, then mix in your chosen color, fragrances, herbs, minerals, or whatever other ingredients you want. Just pour the final mixture into a mold and let it cool for a couple of hours. And as simply as it sounds, once the mixture is completely hardened, it is now ready to be used or sell.

More advanced soap making methods such as the "cold process", "hot process", and "rebatching" will be discuss later on.

Soap Making – A Basic Chemical Reaction

Fundamentally, soap is the product of a basic chemical reaction between essential oils or fats, and "lye".

The primary difference between your Grandmother's greasy, harsh, lye soap and your sumptuous handmade soap is the choice of ingredients and the precision of measurements during the making process.

For better understanding, imagine it this way: You could make a simple bread with just the use of water and flour. Technically it's a bread, but the sad part is that it isn't very tasty or the like. On the other hand, if your bread recipe is made using fresh eggs, yeast, sea salt, a whole-grain flour, and honey, you'll not end up with a simple bread but an exquisite and extra tasty bread.

Of course it's just the same with soap making. By intricately choosing the best quality and combination of essential oils, fragrance, and a lively colorant, I'm sure your soap will most likely become the most ideal soap ever in existence, at least in your area.

NATURAL SOAP

Creating natural soap also means preventing the utilization of various ingredients that might be toxic or are manufactured in many ways that uses suspicious chemicals or techniques. In other words, always avoid using artificial perfumes, dyes, and additives when making soap.

Of course, some individuals might want to attempt creating soap just for fun and enjoyment, and thus aren't really worried about using all natural. The point is that, if you're just going to effort of making your own homemade soap, then why just not create a product that is completely harmless for your friends, family, and yourself?

INGREDIENTS BEHIND SOAP MAKING

You know, most of my friends frequently ask me on how to make a homemade soap. But some are also asking, "What actually is soap?"

For all we know, the main aspect of all soap recipes have basically 2 main ingredients in it, and those are Lye or also known as Sodium Hydroxide and oil and essential oils.

Your homemade soap recipe is just a simple but controlled process. Chemically fused into a new compound and that is the "soap".

Of course, I will share you the top 4 most common process of making soap later on in the book, so stay tuned!

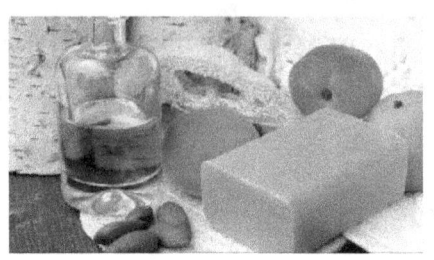

Sodium Hydroxide – Lye

Now, let's talk about what is lye. First and foremost, let me state the fact that you can't really create a soap without this very core ingredient of soap. Many people shy away from creating soap because of the experience with the harsh lye soap that their grandmas' made or perhaps the thought of putting caustic soda into personal care products is somewhat scary.

Well, making soap is fundamentally a chemical reaction between lye which is a base, and essential oils, which are acids. Meaning, when mix together, they will form a complete new material which is gentle and close to neutral in pH.

If you still like to make soap at home but are still a little unsure if you can really handle lye then, I advise you to know the Melt and Pour soap making process. This method uses a pre-made soap that will come in cubes or blocks that you must melt, and just simply pour into moulds. Fret not, because I will also be discussing it because this is one of the 4 processes that I was talking about earlier.

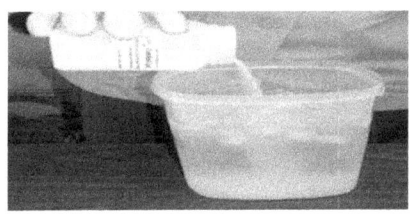

"Sodium Hydroxide a.k.a. Lye"

Water

Water is one of the primary ingredients when making soap because it helps activate the lye and spread over to the oils. But there will probably be no more water left in your homemade soap by the time you use them because the water will evaporate during the 4 to 6 weeks of the curing stage which will make the soap a little smaller and mush harder than we you took them from their moulds.

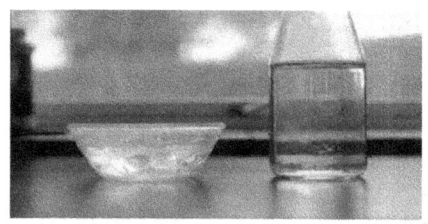

"H_2O a.k.a. Water"

Essential Oils and Fats

You can use any fat or oil to make soap and with your own recipes you can make whenever you want from single oil to a dozen. Though, if you are still a beginner, it is highly recommended that you should just use three to five types of oils. A Castile soap that was made from a single oil can be a little tricky to get used to into making, and picking more oils than necessary can be costly.

From every essential oil that you will utilize to combine with the lye to make a soap trait of that oil and some are chosen to give hardness into the soap bar while other type just provides cleansing, conditioning, and lather. Some examples of most typical oils used in making soap are:

☐ Beeswax

☐ Coconut Oil

☐ Olive Oil

☐ Cocoa Butter

☐ Soybean Oil

☐ Palm Oil

☐ Shea Butter

☐ Almond Oil

1.) Beeswax will provide hardness to your soap and an excellent scent.

2.) Coconut Oil will make your soap hard with many fluffy lather and cleansing properties.

3.) Olive Oil is good for conditioning and excellent for almost all skin types.

4.) Cocoa Butter will give extra moisture and skin protection that also hardens your soap.

5.) Soybean Oil gives a stable lather and provides excellent conditioning for the skin.

6.) Palm Oil is great for making soap but make sure that you consider using oil that has been certified as sustainable.

7.) Shea Butter is quite hard to turn into a typical soap but it's great as a moisturizing soap.

8.)Almond Oil is commonly used because it provides light feeling and excellent moisturizing.

When you are starting to formulate your own recipe, you must choose essential oils that that would make up the totality of your soap recipe, like olive and coconut oil, and those oils that can be used to superfat. If you didn't know, superfatting is the adding of extra essential oils at the end of your soap making process that is free floating instead of combining with lye and transforming it into soap.

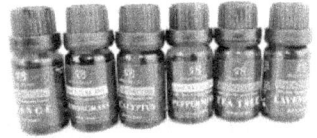

"Essential Oils"

Antioxidants

Preservatives must be only used for wet products because water builds a habitat where germs can harbour. That's why soap, doesn't need preservatives because the water used on the recipe will evaporate.

Though if you are superfatting your recipe, then what you want to add is an antioxidant in order to aid free-floating oils stabilize and prevent rancidity.

There are actually just two primary antioxidants that soap manufacturers use in a very small amount during the end of soap making. Those are:

☐ Grapefruit Seed Extract which is extracted from the seeds of grapefruit. This clear and thick liquid does not give a scent to your soap and is excellent at keeping other oils from getting spoiled.

Rosemary Oleoresin Extract on the other hand is extracted from rosemary leaves as the name implies. It is a little thick and has a powerful smell.

Soap Fragrance – Essential Oils

Others might choose to let their homemade soaps scent speak for themselves and just leave it to smell like clean, simple, and homemade soap.

One way is to utilize essential oils in your recipe like beeswax or sesame because they can impart their own natural and original fragrance.

As for me, I've made an unscented soap that was fragranced with using only natural aroma of oatmeal and guess what? It's quite popular with those individuals suffering from extremely sensitive skin or allergic reactions from fragrance of various kinds.

Also, I just personally love soap that has subtly scented and leaves your skin smells great and gorgeous. Of course, I have used oils for my home made soap from the beginning of my soap making but I've also experimented with just using fragrance oils that are commercially manufactured perfumes for toilets. Obviously, both have their cons and pros though if you like the concept of scent that has therapeutic properties then I highly advice you to stick with using essential oils.

Essential oils have excellent medicinal properties and could help your skin to heal or even clear your airways and your sinus. But the drawback of using essential oils is that their propensity and expense for fading with time if you leave your soap sitting on direct sunlight. This could be very serious for citrus essential oils like oranges and lemons.

On the other hand, unlike essential oils, fragrance oils are quite cheap but still have scents that last for ages, and have much different range to pick from. If you happen to like a baby powder scented shampoo or soap that smells just like coconut then you must use fragrance oils. The drawback of using fragrance oils is that they are patented and have trademarks.

In various cases, fragrance oils are made of allergens and petrochemicals that make people to have skin reactions or sneeze. Using fragrance oils to your homemade soap just simply means that your end product will not be natural anymore.

Know What Scent Fixers Are

From the discussion earlier, I mentioned that the scent of essential oils could fade gradually, but fortunately there are numerous ways to fix the scent in order for them to last longer. Sometimes another essential oils could help other oils to stick and somehow it is ideal to utilize another additive that works to absorb the essential oils on it.

Practically, scent fixers are quite advanced in the field of soap making, but it's good to add them with your experiments to learn more.

Colors

Usually, you have numerous choices for coloring your soap which includes powders you can buy from specific suppliers and even plants and flowers that could be growing in your backyard or garden.

You can also choose oils that will impart a natural color to your soap or just use ingredients what can be gives warm color to the final product.

With that said, here are some natural coloring agents and tips:

☐Choosing Your Oil – some of essential oils like olive oil will give a creamier or yellow color to your soap, while light or white colored oils will give a white homemade soap.

☐ Clays – Clays helps to detox and exfoliate your skin. Though it's limited to just red, pink, white, and green, cosmetic clays can provide additional natural color to your soap.

☐ Micas and Minerals – they are available on a large range of colors that can help you hit most of the color of a rainbow. Remember, that while thsse cosmetic materials are considered intrinsic, they are both made in a laboratory setting. Micas and minerals are found in nature but are usually tainted with unsafe heavy metals, that's why they are not really fitted for use.

☐ Sugars such as honey and milk will caramelise if you add them to your batch just before trace.

☐Roots, Flowers, and Herbs are all natural types of great colors. Use Alkanet root for making purple soaps, Calendula if you want a golden orange soap, and Madder root if you are fond of pink.

Chapter 5: Understanding The Basics

It is important, as a beginner, to understand your ingredients and which blends go well together. Soap needs lather and it needs cleansing properties. It goes without saying and is also critical that it is gentle on the skin. Read on to discover a whole other side of yourself and you may even find your inner apothecary.

Basically, you can invade your pantry in search of some of the basic ingredients.

Avocado oil – check

Sunflower oil – check

Canola (rapeseed) oil – check

Then there's the more traditionally used coconut oil, palm oil and olive oil as a base for many hard soaps. Coconut oil also enriches the texture and creates soapsuds. Oil does not store for long periods of time as it will turn rancid, especially if you live in areas prone to high temperatures.

There's also a move away from palm Oil due to some concerns over Palm oil plantations which threaten the Orang-utan population. It is not a sustainable practice and rain-forests are being destroyed with no hope of restitution. So, take care to use sustainable palm oil or other oils.

There are means of extracting your own essential oils and there are ways of combining hard fat or lard in creating your soap masterpiece. This however is time consuming and it would be wise to learn a little more about the craft first before going to these lengths.

Lye is a product, available as flakes, a coarse powder or even as a solution. It is readily available in pharmacies and some supermarkets. Essentially, lye when mixed with water, followed by oils, fats and fragrances combines to create a gradual chemical reaction. Soap is the result.

Essential oils are the key to any good soap and are natural ingredients. They represent the heart of any plant and are extracted from various parts of the plant through different methods. Due to the pain-staking process, they are expensive and so, be sure to use them sparingly.

Eucalyptus essential oil will cure your blocked nose in a jiffy and has a very strong smell so needs to be tempered by other sweeter smells when it is used in soap. Good combinations include Rosemary, Cedarwood and Lemon Grass.

Peppermint essential oil is another strong one and blends well with grapefruit, lemon, and other citrus oils.

Rosemary essential oil goes well with Cinnamon and Citronella. Another strong one.

Lavender oil is an old favourite as Lavender is known to aid sleep, reduce anxiety and has even been used to treat tension headaches when it is inhaled. It also reduces irritation after stings and insect bites.

Sweet Orange blends well with lavender and spice oils such as Cinnamon.

Apart from essential oils, you can add fragrance oils although they are not all natural and may be part natural and part synthetic. You can also add flowers and seeds, herbs and even oats and some spices.

Chapter 6: 3 Soap Making Techniques

Even though you have total control of the ingredients that go into your soap, you need to have the right technique to turn your soap recipes to reality. Here are 3 soap making techniques that you can try out to make your own batch of soap.

1. Melt and pour

The melt and pour technique is the easiest for beginner soap makers. It requires using a premade base that already went through the process of saponification. All you have to do is choose a soap base that you want to use (olive, goat's milk, aloe vera, clear glycerin), melt it down, and add your ingredients like colorants, scents, herbs and exfoliants. The best part about using the melt and pour method is that you can quickly produce a batch within 24 hours.

This is the best technique to use if you want to make soap to give away as gifts, or if you're worried about exposing yourself to lye. Most of the recipes you'll find in this ebook makes use of the melt and pour technique because it's also a good way to gain some confidence before you move on to soap making from scratch.

Benefits of melt and pour soap

Melt and pour soap can be a good project to do with children because it's relatively safe. This is also perfect for those who are still nervous about exposing themselves to lye.

While some advanced soap makers will argue that the melt and pour soap isn't really soap making, it makes for a good entry way. When I was first starting out, it was melt and pour that motivated me to try out the cold process.

Nowadays, there is a wide range of different melt and pour bases you can choose from so your soap making possibilities are endless. But be careful because some soap bases may contain parabens and petroleum. Make sure to check the label for ingredients before buying your soap base.

2. Cold process

The cold process method is what I like to call the traditional way to make soap. It involves mixing lye with oils and requires a curing time for the soap to set. Many soap makers prefer the cold process because it allows them to fully customize their soap. It gives them complete freedom to choose and control the ingredients that will go into the batch. It's purposeful soap making because every ingredient has a very specific purpose and reason for being in the soap recipe. This is the technique for you if you want to customize not just the scent of your soap, but also the oils that go in it.

Just a word of caution though. Making cold process soap can yield unpredictable results. But that's just all part of the learning process. You'll find some easy cold process recipes in this ebook to try once you feel more confident to take the next step. To give you an idea on how it's done, here's a short gist of the cold process.

The Gist of the Cold Process

Pour lye into water and never vice versa. If you do it the other way around, expect a dangerous explosion to happen. After you've mixed the lye with the water, give the solution time to cool.

Always melt solid oils before mixing the oils you're going to use together. Before combining the lye solution with your oils, make sure that they're already cooled to around 120 degrees Fahrenheit.

Mix the lye solution with the oils until you see a trace. A trace is basically the point where if you drip soap, you'll see a line form on top. This is a signal that the saponification process is beginning.

You can now add your chosen additives like essential oils, colorants, and dried herbs and flowers.

Once you're happy with your soap batch, it's time to pour it into your chosen mold. To stabilize the temperature of your soap and make sure that it doesn't turn cold immediately, especially during the winter months, wrap the mold with a towel or blanket for added insulation.

Allow the soap to dry for at least 24 hours before you cut it into bars. Then set aside to cure.

It takes around 4-5 weeks for cold process soap to cure. Remember to flip your soap bars every week so that they evenly cure.

Allow your soap to go through the saponification process as it cures. Over the next weeks you can expect the soap to harden. If you don't let the soap cure, your soap will immediately melt when exposed to water. The longer the saponification process, the better your homemade soap will be to your skin.

3. Hot process

The hot process is the hardest soap making technique of them all. It involves heating the lye and oils as they mix together. While exposing these ingredients to heat can speed up the saponification process, it's can also be very volatile. Even more volatile than the cold process. Many soap makers consider this method to be the ultimate technique because of the shorter curing time. But it can also be very labor intensive. I've decided to not include the hot process in this ebook because it's not beginner friendly.

Basic Soap Making Ingredients and Equipment

To get started on your first batch of homemade soap, it's important that you avoid using ingredients that could be toxic to your health. Steer clear of artificial additives like dyes and perfumes and invest in high quality and organic ingredients. Remember, your soap is only as good as the ingredients that you put in it. If you're unsure of how an ingredient was made or where it came from, it's best to look for all-natural alternatives instead. You're already putting in a lot of effort into handcrafting your soap. You might as well use the best ingredients your money can buy.

INGREDIENTS:

Most people think that you need special knowledge in chemistry to make soap. But as long as you have basic math skills and you can follow directions, you can come up with your own batch of homemade soap in no time. Before we dive into the process, let's first look at the ingredients you'll need to make soap in your own home.

- Sodium Hydroxide/Lye

Sodium hydroxide or lye, is one of the two basic components of soap. Without it, the saponification process can't happen. While many people tend to shy away from this ingredient, there's no avoiding it in the soap making process. If you're making soap for the first time and you feel a bit hesitant to use lye, don't worry. I recommend that you start off with a 'melt and pour' soap base and build your soap recipe from there.

The Melt and pour option takes away the guesswork in soap making by giving you the option to use a premade soap base. Simply cut into small chunks, melt everything in the microwave, and customize it by adding your own blend of different ingredients. Most of the recipes you'll read in this book makes use of melt and pour soap so you won't have to worry about handling lye.

- Oils and Fats

The other basic component of soap is oils or fats. You can use just about any type of oil or fat to make soap. You can even mix and match different oils to match your skin type. But if you're just starting out, it's best to keep it simple. Each oil has its own purpose in soap making. There are some that makes soap hard while there are others, when combined, give soap its lather. There are also those that cleanse better than others, or keeps skin moisturized and bouncy. Since most of the recipes you'll find in this ebook are melt and pour based, you can easily choose a base that you think would work best for the soap you want to create. Just to give you an idea, here are a few types of oils you can use to make soap:

Coconut oil - the most common oil used in soap making. Known for its cleansing properties and contributes to the hardness of a soap. Great for making fluffy lathery soaps.

Olive oil - one of the most popular oils that many DIY soap makers swear by. Rich in Vitamin K and vitamin E, and makes for a creamy type of soap. Very good for moisturizing and conditioning all skin types.

Palm oil - although it can be very tricky to use, this oil is great for making lathery soap. Doesn't spoil easily so it helps soap last longer. Add this to your soap mix if you want a hard bar. Choose palm oil that was harvested properly and responsibly.

Castor oil - acts as a humectant so it's great for moisturizing bars. Draws moisture from the air into the skin. Very similar to beeswax but relatively more affordable. Add castor oil to your soap mix if you want added lather.

Cocoa butter - offers skin protection. Soap makers use this to harden soap and provide moisturizing properties. Can be comedogenic so avoid using in facial soaps.

Shea butter - can be difficult to use since it can give soap a buttery feel. Great for moisturizing and nourishing skin. If you want to make a shea butter soap, use a melt and pour base instead of creating it from scratch. A melt and pour base makes it more manageable.

Sweet almond oil - soap makers use this to make a lighter soap. Doesn't feel heavy on the skin but conditions and moisturizes like nothing else.

Lard/tallow - great for creating a creamy and hard bar of soap. It hardens to a white colored soap that most people grew up with. Add lard or tallow to your soap recipe if you want to make a traditional bar.

- Water

Water is an important ingredient because it activates lye and disperses it to the oils. Water in soap naturally evaporates during the curing process, leaving soap bars harder and smaller than when they were first taken out of the molds.

- Essential oils

Essential oils are what will make your batch of natural soap unique. You can customize your blend depending on the properties you want your soap to have. Because there's a wide range of essential oils readily available to you, you can pick and choose according to what's in season and your budget. This is where the fun in soap making begins. As long as you can apply the essential oil topically, you can add it to your soap. The only problem with using essential oil is that its scent can easily fade when exposed to direct sunlight. Just make sure to store your soap in a cool dry place. Here are a few of the best essential oils to add to your soap:

Lavender - acts as an antiseptic. Calms and relaxes the senses. Has a herbaceous floral scent.

Rose - has anti-inflammatory properties and treats redness. Moisturizes dry skin. Has a floral scent.

Tea tree - has antifungal and antibacterial properties. Popularly used for treating acne. Has an antiseptic and resinous scent.

Lemon - acts as an antiseptic. Whitens dark spots. Has a fresh citrusy scent.

Sweet orange - has skin toning properties. Relaxes the spirit. Has a fruity citrusy scent.

Rosemary - acts as an astringent. Stimulates skin cell growth. Has a camphorous herbal scent.

Peppermint - stimulates skin turnover. Cooling to the skin. Offers pain relief. Has a minty herbal scent.

Cedarwood - has antiseptic and astringent properties. Improves skin tone. Has a woody masculine scent.

Clary sage - Relaxes and calms the spirit. Balances sebum production. Has a sweet floral scent.

Patchouli - regenerates skin cells and promotes skin turnover. Can be used as a deodorant. Has an exotic earthy scent.

- Fragrance oil

Fragrance oils are relatively cheaper than essential oils and they last much longer. While many soap makers rely on fragrance oils to add oomph to their soap creations, these oils may contain allergens and petrochemicals that can cause skin reactions. Check the labels and make sure to choose organic.

- Clays

Clays come in different colors so you can use this to give your soap creations added drama. Clay can also act as a light exfoliant and detox the skin. Bentonite clay, in particular, can unclog pores of toxins and also help lighten scars. It can heal skin by reducing redness and inflammation.

- Exfoliants

Exfoliants like ground almonds, ground rice, and rolled oats can be added to your soap mix if you want a soap that can effectively scrub skin. These natural exfoliants promote fast skin turnover without using harmful chemicals.

- Mica powdered pigments

Mica powdered pigments are available in a wide array of colors that you can recreate the rainbow in your soap creations. While these pigments are sourced naturally, some brands may mix them with heavy metals to produce specific hues. Again, do your own research before you choose a brand. You want your powdered pigments to be safe as possible.

- Flowers and herbs

Dried flowers and herbs are used not just for decorating, but also for tinting soaps. You can mix flowers and herbs in some oil to coax out some color and scent. A popular way to use dried flowers and herbs is to add them on top of newly poured soap before it dries. Dried flower petals tend to lose its color when exposed to high heat so add them only when the soap has slightly cooled.

EQUIPMENT:

One reason why many people get into soap making is because you don't necessarily need to buy new equipment to get started. Just take a look around your kitchen and you probably already have the basics. An old pan, some spoons, old cups, a couple of plastic bowls, a stove or microwave, and you're all set.

There's no need to take out a loan or max out your credit card to start making soap. And while I highly suggest that you use what you already have, make sure that you can afford to dedicate your equipment for this purpose. You don't want anyone in your family eating salad from a bowl that you used to mix lye earlier. Even if you use natural ingredients to make your soap, there's still a bit of chemistry involved so do be careful. Here's a quick rundown of equipment you'll need to make soap in your kitchen.

- Soap molds

It's easy to find soap molds in all shapes and sizes. If you're going to invest in a couple, make sure that they're silicone because they don't require much prepping. It's easy to pop the soap out of the silicone molds because they're so flexible. If you're taking the traditional route and using wooden boxes as molds, line them first with wax paper before pouring in your soap mix. This way, it won't be much of a struggle to get the soap out.

- Measuring equipment (cups, spoons, digital scale)

You need measuring equipment like cups and spoons, and a digital scale for when you start working with lye, to measure your ingredients. While cups and spoons are perfectly okay for melt and pour recipes, you'll need to be a bit more precise when it comes to making cold process soaps. This is when a digital kitchen scale will come in handy. When making soap from scratch, you'll need to measure your ingredients by weight before you start working to avoid catastrophic results.

- Steel whisk or a stick blender

You'll also need something to mix all your ingredients together. If you're making soap with a melt and pour base, a steel whisk will suffice. But if you're navigating your way around lye and oils, then you definitely need a stick blender to make sure that your ingredients come together to make a good batch of soap.

- Silicone spatula

Just like in baking, there's nothing quite like a silicone spatula to get as much batter or soap as possible out of your bowl or pan. Trust me, this is one of the most underrated kitchen equipment.

- Goggles and gloves

Always remember: Safety first. Always make sure that you have a pair of goggles and gloves in your work area before getting started. And even though soap making isn't actually seen as a very dangerous activity, making soap from scratch will involve handling chemically volatile ingredients. Lye can be very dangerous as it is considered a highly alkaline substance. If you're not careful, it can burn skin and cause serious damage to property.

- Mixing bowls

Mixing bowls and containers are pretty much self-explanatory, but make sure that you use bowls and containers that are designed to take on high heat. If you're going to use metal bowls and containers, opt for stainless steel as other metals have the tendency to react adversely with lye and soap in general. As a rule of thumb, anything that comes into contact with lye from then on should only be used for soap making purposes only.

Chapter 7: Soap Making For Boredom

Is it true that you are feeling kind of level and exhausted requiring something to possess your interests? Tired of playing web amusements for a considerable length of time and no enthusiasm for anything on TV? Side benefits can be the solution for your situation; it surely was the response for me. My fundamental issue is that I need to do it all, I need to attempt each art and side interest I keep running over!

Some diversions can fill a double need by furnishing you with good pay from your interest. Making cleansers and shower salts is a leisure activity that can be sheltered, modest and enthralling... also it can pay for itself if you offer your completed items.

I am going to furnish you with orderly direction alongside formulas for things that you can make and use to finish your home, give as endowments or even offer a benefit.

To discover what cleanser making includes, begin necessarily by starting with a simple formula, Chocolate soap is a decent starter and here is the thing that you require:

12 oz ground cleanser

5 oz water

1/4 glass moment cocoa powder

1/8 oz Chocolate Scent oil

Join your ground cleanser and water in a pot and set on medium warmth; When the soap has dissolved the consolidated cocoa powder and chocolate scent; Blend well and after that pack into molds and permit to sit until totally solidified.

When you are prepared stride it up we will start with making glycerine cleansers... this is the thing that you should make Apple Tart Cleanser:

4oz. Clear, Unscented Glycerine Cleanser

1 Tablespoon Fluid Cleanser

One teaspoon Fluid Glycerine

1/2 teaspoon Apple Scent Oil

2 Drops Red Sustenance Shading

1/2 teaspoon Ground Cinnamon

To begin with you dissolve cleanser in little container over low warmth or in a glass in the microwave; Include Fluid Cleanser and glycerine and mix tenderly however well; Include scent and/or shading; Include cinnamon and mix; Permit to remain for several minutes, sufficiently only to begin to thicken so when you combine the cinnamon again will be all the more equitably disseminated; Fill molds. Permit to set totally (in or out of cooler). At the point when totally set you can wrap your cleanser in plastic wrap, sweet cellophane packs likewise work exceptionally well.

Another kind of glycerin cleanser that is intriguing to make is Apricot Freesia, and this is the thing that you will require:

1 lb White Glycerin Cleanser Base

12 Drops Astronomical Shading Canary Yellow

11 Drops Astronomical Shading Red

One t. Apricot Freesia FO

Elements For "Whipped Cream" Topping:

4 oz White Glycerin Cleanser Base

¼ t. Apricot Freesia FO

Initially you soften cleanser base for tart in a twofold heater; After it is totally dissolved, include shading and scent;

Empty blend into a biscuit tin and permit to solidify; Expel from tin; Melt cleanser base for fixing and include a shake of Shimmer Dust; Utilizing an electric blender, blend until thickened and bubbly; Shower with rubbing liquor and spoon the fixing onto the tarts and permit a portion of the garnish to keep running over sides; Top with a dash of Shimmer Dust (discretionary)

Being one who does a ton of stimulating and investing energy with youngsters, Treat Cutter Cleanser was an absolute necessity! The making of this cleanser obliges one to be inventively free and is a decent specialty for children, with grown-up supervision obviously.

Dissolve and Pour cleanser base(opaque)

Fragrance (discretionary)

Shading (must be fluid, similar to gels)

treat sheet (must have no less than a 1/2 in. edge on it)

blade (to twirl your hues!)

treat cutters

In the first place you will need to liquefy down the cleanser base and aromas; You can give the principle support a shading in the event that you wish or abandon it white; Pour the base on the treated sheet and include hues and twirl every one of them over - this is the place you get the chance to be innovative! When this dries, pop the piece of cleanser out of the treated sheet. Use handle cutters to cut up the soap.

There are bunches of various things you can do with this for the case you can make...

Christmas Cleanser: Whirl red and green into white and utilize treat cutters;

Sweet Stick Cleanser: Twirl red into white with peppermint aroma and treat stick cutters;

Easter/Spring: Whirl various pastels and discover some fun treat cutters;

fourth of July: Devoted white cleanser with a beautiful red and blue twirl (locate a decent star cutter!)

So you see your alternatives are boundless to the extent what you can make and offer if you seek!

Chapter 8: Safety Procedures: Working With Alkali

You should remember that alkali is a dangerous active substance. In dry form alkali is not too active, but it is highly soluble in water, thus there is plenty of heat. You should take into consideration that existing water is fairly too much to react even on dry skin, let alone the fact about the mucous membranes. Chemical burns can arouse on the skin and mucous alkali, in case of inhaling vapors and aerosols caustic, irritation of the upper respiratory tract can be noted, severe pain develops due to the contact with caustic alkali in esophagus and stomach, blood vomiting, painful shock.

Remember that the presence of children and animals while working with alkali is unacceptable!

It sounds, of course, threatening, therefore there are special safety rules, so in order not to hurt yourselves and others, but also to create a perfect product for your health and beauty. Working with alkali one should take into consideration the consequences. The rules are simple and are logically followed from the possible affecting effects of alkali:

• Protect eyes with the help of glasses!

• Protect respiratory organs with respirator!

• Protect skin covering with clothes, apron and gloves, and hair with a cap or a scarf!

Besides, when working with alkali you should follow certain rules, hence you can avoid all unpleasant consequences:

1. Pour alkali into the water but not vice versa. Then gradually add caustic, stirring constantly, and step by step increase the concentration of the alkaline solution. If

you do the opposite and add water to the alkali, there will be a rough chemical reaction with the high heat and alkali vapors.

2. The fluid for alkaline solution should be well chilled. It will be better if you freeze it to icy condition. Then you are more likely to be able to avoid alkali vapor emissions at its dissolution. If you use non-frozen liquid, then it may boil, emitting corrosive vapor in the result of chemical reaction.

3. Do not lean over the pot containing liquid when stirring alkali. It is better to keep your hands far away, hence the vapor will not harm you.

4. In order to avoid the risk of tipping over the pot with liquid while stirring, it is better to put it in the sink and let cold water cools down the liquid.

5. The room where you work should be well ventilated: open the window, or you can also turn on the draught system.

If alkaline liquid still got on your skin, the most important is - DO NOT PANIC, place the affected area under the running water and treat it with vinegar or lemon juice (keep them not far away). Alkali neutralizes acid, and you will avoid unpleasant consequences. If dry alkali got on your skin, it is better to wash it without using water, and then treat the skin with vinegar. Experience will come to you along with practice, and you will develop an optimal course of actions. To begin with, I can advise the following:

1. Make the recipe for your soap.

2. Measure the necessary amount of oil (it is preferable to place liquid and solid oil in different containers.)

3. Weigh liquid (ice) according to the recipe.

4. Measure additional useful components and oil for superfat.

5. Put solid oils, waxes to melt over the water bath.

6. Wear protective equipment (glasses, respirator, apron, gloves).

7. Weigh alkali in a glass or plastic container (you can use sour cream, yogurt disposable plastic cups or containers).

8. Put the container with ice into the sink and turn on cold water.

9. Pour alkali on the ice, stirring constantly. Ice will start to melt immediately.

10. After complete dissolution of the alkali liquid, pour the liquid into the oil mixture through a strainer (plastic or stainless steel). Then mix it.

Soap making terms & equipment

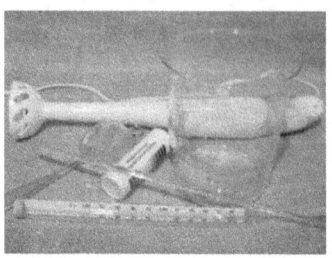

It is better to allocate to pick out a special dish for soap making and not use it anymore for cooking.

So, we need the following equipment:

• a glass pan, steel or enameled aluminum – to mix all components;

• a larger diameter pan - for water bath;

• a container made of glass or plastic that can withstand high temperature (at least 100 ° C) - to prepare alkaline liquid in (mixing caustic with liquid, a high heat chemical reaction occurs with high heat up to boiling of the liquid, hence you should use a sufficiently large pot to avoid splashing of the liquid). It is better to use special laboratory glassware for these purposes: heat-resistant glass beaker.

• a glass spoon or a glass stick, porcelain or plastic - to mix alkaline liquid;

• a plastic container (disposable) to weighing alkali;

• two thermometers (one to measure the oil temperature, the second to measure alkali liquid);

• strainer made of plastic or stainless steel to strain alkaline liquid (gauze will also do);

• scales with the division of 1 g, in case if you want to cook at least 0.3 kg of soap; to make soap with less than 300 g, use more accurate scale(0.1 g);

• hand blender - to mix all components;

• test strips to measure pH;

• plastic or steel spoon to stir the liquid;

- a mold for soap if you make soap by cutting, it is very convenient to use a special wooden box or silicone-loaf shape, but if they are not suitable, use plastic food storage containers, cartons of juice, etc. For a batch of soap you can use silicone molds or again take out some packaging products: yogurt, cream, curds, cakes, molds for children's sandboxes, etc.

- towels or dense fabric to wrap soap.

Do not forget about safety rules too:

- apron;

- gloves;

- protective mask (respirator);

- Protective glasses;

- hair beanie;

- vinegar liquid or lemon juice in case if alkaline liquid gets on your skin.

Let's once again emphasize that only stainless steel, enamel (no chips), glass (heat resistant), plastic or silicone utensils and tools are allowed to use. NEVER use utensils made of aluminum or other metals prone to oxidation, because they can interact with alkali.

Types of oils and their properties

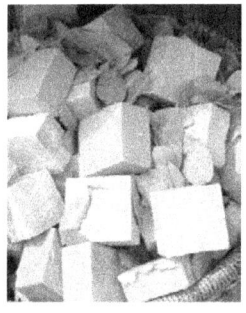

To make natural soap by yourself three main ingredients are needed: alkali, water, fats. Fats are the basis products to make soap, both vegetable and of animal origin. Vegetable oils are divided into liquid and solid. Liquid vegetable oil, is also known as fundamental or transmitting, since it serves as the fundament (base) to dilute essential oils and to transfer their useful constituents on your skin. Solid vegetable oils otherwise are called butters (e.g., shea oil), some oil belongs to semi-solid or soft oil for its consistency (e.g., coconut oil). All vegetable oils have a certain therapeutic properties, they include vitamins, minerals and other nutrients.

One of the advantages of making natural soaps is that you can make soap by yourselves with individual properties- nutrient or moisturizing, cleansing or healing etc. You should know the properties of oils used in soap making much better.

Soaps can be welded both with one type of oil and a mixture of vegetable and animal fats. These are the most popular types of monosoaps (using one type of oil):

- castile soap: the classic type of this soap is brewed with 100% olive oil which was ripened at least six months. This soap is like a fine wine, the longer it ripens the better it gets. Castile soap is a very delicate, and is suitable for all skin types, especially for sensitive and allergy-prone. It is so gentle that it can be used for babies;

- palm soaps: brewed from palm oil, this soap is very economic and has little foam;

- coconut soaps: made with coconut oil, makes much foam, it is also known as sailors' soap as it can foam in cold sea water, but it can dry the skin;

- soap from shea oil: a truly luxurious soap which lets the skin feel cleansed without drying it.

However, not all vegetable oils are able to create balanced, in all respects, soap, hence a mixture of oils is often used. Each oil is responsible for certain properties and physical characteristics of the future soap: color, hardness, ductility, foaming, cleansing, conditioning effect, etc. Making soap recipe all these properties should be taken into account.

First you need to decide on the oils, which will be the basis, the foundation for your soaps. Logically, the solid oils (butters) will be responsible mainly for the hardness of soap, and liquid vegetable oils – for conditioning and caring properties.

Usually the following formula is used to make a balanced soap:

- 60% of all oils should be composed of oils, responsible for the hardness of soap (palm, coconut, palm kernel, babassu, mango oil, shea oil);

- 25% - oils making foam (castor, coconut, palm, palm kernel, babassu, olive oil);

- 15% - oils with conditioning and caring properties (almond oil, avocado oil, shea oil, mango oil, cocoa oil, grape seed oil, jojoba oil, apricot seeds, macadamia oil, etc.).

First soap must perform its primary function: cleansing, hence making natural soap oils are generally included into the consistency of natural soaps. These oils / fats include (in descending order of cleansing properties) murumuru oil (73), babassu (70), coconut (67) palm (65) oil, goat fat (16), ghee (clarified butter) (15), butter (15) and mutton tallow (14), tallow (8). Oil which is responsible for cleansing, promotes much foaming in soap. If their total amount is more than 30%, the soap may parch skin.

The concept of superfat is also used in soap making. These are oils that will not react with alkali, and retaining all its useful properties, give them caring, softening, moisturizing additives. Depending on the type of soap the superfat percentage ranges from 0 to 15%. For example, making soap for normal skin another 5-8% of the caring oil of the major oils' total weight is added, and for very dry skin the superfat percentage may reach up to 15%.

Below is a list of the most popular vegetable oils and animal fats with their properties used in soap making:

• oil of apricot pits: used in the soap as a powerful caring supplement for mature and sensitive skin, with 5-10% percentage of input.

• avocado oil: moisturizing soap for dry skin. In combination with olive oil this soap will be great for kids. Use up to 15% in recipes.

• babassu oil: a perfect moisturizer for all skin types. Kernel oil has similar properties with coconut and palm oils: it increases the foaming, gives the soap hardness. Percentage of input - up to 30%. If other foaming oils are used in soap (coconut), then try to keep the total number not more than 30% as far as it can dry the skin instead of caring.

• grape seed oil: is used as an additive in a moisturizing soap, input- 5%.

• beef tallow: allows you to get a very solid snow white soap. It gives a low, stable foaming. It has moisturizing property. It goes well with coconut and olive oil. Classical soap content - up to 40%.

• walnut oil: has excellent moisturizing and emollient properties, but has poor foaming properties, use up to 10%.

• jojoba oil: soap with moisturizing and soothing properties, suitable for young and sensitive skin. Provides stable foaming, speeds up the "trace". 5% is enough in the recipe.

• wheat germ oil: it is rich in vitamin E, a natural preservative, nourishes dry, damaged and mature skin. Recommended maximum quantity of usage is 10-15% in recipes.

• cocoa oil: adds chocolate flavor to the soap and has softening, healing properties. Gives the soap hardness and fragility at the same time, so do not use more than 10-15% in combination with soft oils, otherwise the soap will crumble. Stable foaming, creamy.

• castor oil: moisturizes, rich in saturated acids, capable of keeping liquids, it turns to be emollient soap with abundant creamy foam. It does not harden. Speeds up the appearance of a "trace". Use up to 20%.

• coconut oil: very hard soap with large fluffy but unstable foaming. Gives cleansing and whitening properties to the soap. Add up to 15-30% coconut oil to the soap of every day usage, otherwise it will dry the skin because of its high cleansing properties. Soap for hard salted water usage - up to 100%.

• hemp oil: light silky foam, moisturizing properties, soothes the skin, prevents neurodermatis. Makes the soap soft, so is widely used in making liquid soap. Soap has little expiration date. Therefore, it is better to add vitamin E to the composition of such soaps, and keep it in the refrigerator for 3 months. Use up to 10-15% in the recipe.

• sesame oil: has excellent moisturizing and conditioning properties. Distinct characteristic smell of the oil is kept in the soap, so many people use a very small percentage of its input.

• macadamia oil: moisturizing and nourishing properties of this oil is the best fit for a child's sensitive skin as it is hypoallergenic. It is used in soaps as superfatting component.

- mango oil: has a strong moisturizing effect, used for different skin types. When added to soap, oil neutralizes its drying effect on the skin. Soap with mango oil turns to be solid with stable foaming. Percentage of input- 5-15%. Use it in the major compound of soap or add to the mark as superfat.

- sweet almond oil: has excellent skin moisturizing and softening effect. Provides soap with snow white properties. Typical input percentage is 5-10%. It can be used as one of the main components in the soap recipe. Soap made from 100% almond is very pleasant, but it is better to use it in combination with olive and palm oils.

- neem oil (neem) oil is used in soap making for thousands of years to give it some medical properties. Soap with Neem oil has antiseptic, antibacterial, antiviral properties, is an excellent care for skin and produces stable foam. The percentage of input is up to 20%.

• sea buckthorn oil: soap with wound-healing properties. Usage is up to 5%.

• olive oil: it turns to be pleasant, delicate, soothing with silky foam.

• palm oil: it foams well, solid, slowly soluble in water. This soap has long expiration date. Use up to 100% in recipes.

• palm kernel oil: it gives the necessary flexibility to the soap, whiteness, prevents cracking and provides good foaming and gentle but effective cleansing. Use up to 100% in the recipe.

• sunflower oil: light oil, suitable for dry, thin skin. It foams poorly, so it is used in conjunction with soapy oils. It makes light foam with huge bubbles. Limit the amount to 15% to make the soap hard.

- rapeseed oil: it nourishes the skin gently and makes it more supple. It gives silky soft foaming to soap. It is also good as shampoo soap. It reduces the rate of "trace" occurrence, hence it is used in the soap manufacture with complex swirl. Percentage of input: up to 20%.

- lard: solid white soap, stable creamy foaming. Soap turns to be very gentle. Disadvantage: low cleansing property. Typical input percentage- 30-40%.

- pumpkin seed oil: black oil with sunflower seeds smell that gives the soap color (green to deep restrained honey-brown). Percentage input 5-10%.

- shea oil: moisturizing and delicate oil, gives the soap silkiness. Percentage input is up to 10%. However, according to the practice the more there is the shea oil soap, the more pleasant the soap is to the skin. An excellent result shows the usage of 15-30% of shea oil.

- rosehip oil: reduces scarring and promotes skin healing, it is suitable for sensitive skin. With 5- 10% of dosage.

Drawing up the recipe for soap it is also important to note that some of the oil burns out. Soap with such oils deteriorate faster, it may get stained, get some unpleasant smell. Among these oils there are sunflower, walnut oil, linseed oil, corn oil, lard, hazelnut oil. Soap, which is composed of burning oil, must be quickly used.

Olive, jojoba, cocoa, palm oil, coconut oil, palm kernel oil poppy soybean are not spoilt for a long time.

Each oil differs with the acids composition, which react with alkali in different ways. Special programs called soap calculators are used to make recipe. They can give out the needed amount of alkali and liquid to soap the particular type of oil.

Chapter 9: What Is Soap Made From?

Most human beings inquire from people about ways to make cleaning soap but maybe the first question that need to be asked is 'What is Soap'? At the heart of all cleaning soap recipes are two primary elements: oil and lye, additionally acknowledged by its chemical called Sodium Hydroxide. Your soap making recipe will, via an easy however managed process, chemically bond those two elements into a brand new compound – Soap!

The beneath is most effective intended as a creation for your options and every phase may be elevated upon with enough facts to actually fill books.

Lye / Sodium Hydroxide

Right, start from lye. I'd like to start by saying that you simply cannot make your very own soap without lye. A lot of human beings turn away from making soap because of enjoy with the cruel lye soap their grandmothers made or because the idea of placing caustic soda into private care products scares or places them off.

As I shared above, soap making is basically the chemical response among oils, which might be acids, and lye, which is a base. Together they will form a completely new fabric so as to be mild and almost neutral in PH.

If you'd want to make soap however are nonetheless you are feeling a bit unsure approximately handling Sodium Hydroxide then I'd advice that you inspect shopping 'Melt-and-Pour' cleaning soap. It's pre-made soap that you melt, upload extra substances and fragrance, after which pour into molds.

Water

You use water in cleaning soap making to activate the lye and disperse it via the oils. Most of this water evaporates out of your bars at some point of the curing system. That means that your completed bars might be barely smaller than even as you first took them out of their molds.

As a beginner, use the water amount proven inside the cleaning soap recipe you're about to use. This will normally be formulated to give you a 33-38% lye awareness. As you get greater skilled you can water bargain your soap batches however I don't advise you do that at the beginning. Trace time can accelerate and the coloration of the soap may also vary from what you expect.

Oils & Fats

You can use any oil or fats to make soap. Most soap recipes encompass 3-6 oils however some have lots extra, or less.

Soaps made from a single oil, including castile (olive oil) cleaning soap are unusual due to the fact very few unmarried oils make a very good soap. Different oils provide one-of-a-kind homes to soap including hardness, lather, creaminess, and conditioning.

Most soap recipes also are awesome-fatted. This way including more oils on the very cease of the soap making procedure in order to be free-floating for your bars. These extra oils don't combine with lye and makes the difference between a bar of soap that's cleansing and a bar of cleaning soap that's cleaning and moisturizing.

If you're a newbie, please stick with the use of attempted and tested recipes. Common oils utilized in cleaning soap making

•Beeswax — Beeswax Vegetarian however not Vegan, this wax will add hardness in your soap and a beautiful fragrance. Use handiest small amounts of beeswax on your recipes because it stops lathering at larger portions.

•Cocoa Butter – Organic Cocoa Butter gives fantastic moisture and skin protection and additionally allows to harden your cleaning soap. Use in smaller possibilities as a 'superfatting' oil.

•Coconut oil – Coconut Oil creates a difficult bar with hundreds of fluffy lather and cleaning energy.

•Olive oil – Olive oil Pomace cleaning soap made with olive oil is touchy, conditioning, and extraordinary for all skin sorts.

•Palm oil – Palm Oil a brilliant oil for soap making but one this is very arguable. Palm plantations in south-east Asia have caused devastating deforestation and loss of habitat for animals which include Orangutans. If you pick to apply Palm oil please don't forget the use of oil that's been certified as sustainable and attempt to study extra about in which precisely its being grown and who grows them.

•Soybean oil – Soybean oil facilitates create a conditioning bar with a stable lather

•Shea Butter – Shea Butter An exciting oil because it has greater difficulty turning into soap than different oils and will frequently live in your soap as moisturizing butter instead of cleaning soap. Use in smaller chances as a 'superfatting' oil.

•Sweet Almond oil – Sweet Almond Oil used for its mild feeling and capacity to moisturize and condition the skin. Use in smaller probabilities as a 'top notch-fatting' oil.

Chapter 10: Why Should You Make Your Own Soap?

Soap sold commercially is most often made on a large scale with the most cost effective way possible. This includes using chemical detergents, hardening material and other chemicals that are very harmful to your skin. The chemicals in commercial soap often leave your hands dry as they focus on cleaning and forget about pampering your skin. When you make homemade soap, it is made with natural ingredients such as lye and natural oils. Moreover, you can also control what you add in there, for example, adding natural aromatherapy oils or compounds such as glycerin. Glycerin is a small amino acid that is very good for the softness of your skin. The process of soap making naturally produces glycerin. However, most commercial soaps don't have glycerin. That is because they extract it to make use of it for other skin loving and high-quality products such as moisturizing lotions. This leaves the soap hard and irritating to the skin, although it cleans well. But soap also needs to be skin loving and soft on the skin. With natural homemade soap, you can add glycerin or whatever skin friendly ingredient you want to add.

You may argue that homemade soap uses lye and you don't want lye on your skin. The wonder of chemistry is that during the process of saponification, the lye completely dissolves and reacts with the oils used to form soap, and no more lye remains if you have used the correct proportions.

One of the best advantages of making your own soap is that you can be sure of all the ingredients included. You are 100% in control. You can choose to use all-natural products, even the coloring can be used from natural and skin friendly alternatives.

Another beauty of making your own soap is that you are the master of the process. You can control how you want your soap to feel. Do you want to make it soft or hard? What scent do you want your soap to have? Do you want your soap to be frothy and lathery or have little lather? All this you can control by adjusting the proportions of lye and the type of oils you use. For example, using castor oil gives you different results than when using olive oil and so on and so forth. The possibilities are almost endless with homemade soap. Think of all the experimenting fun you can have!

Soap making can be a life changing activity. DIY soap is a fun and relaxing activity to do to release stress. Therefore, it is a great outlet to de-stress and try something new. It is also an outlet to feel different or discover a new hobby. It is a great opportunity to express and discover your creativity by experimenting with different proportions, ingredients and add ons. Moreover, you can always get creative with the shapes of the molds, color combinations, petal additions and even the final packaging. It would also be perfect as a bonding arts and crafts activity. Your homemade soap will make you feel proud about your achievement and progress as you can see your bathroom shelves stacked with the magical work of your hands.

Soap making can also be your chance to increase your income as you can make handmade soap and sell it, making your own brand by using your own creative touch. Homemade soap has helped a lot of females take care of their families by selling the soap they make. Moreover, it is a creative and a wonderful sensual gift to give your friends, family or loved ones. There are tons of reasons to make your own soap, without further ado, let's get into HOW you can make your own soap. But before that, as always, safety first, so let us discuss some safety considerations while making soap at home.

The Benefits of Soap Making

It protects your skin!

I love reading labels on food, and it is no different with products I put onto my body. As it turns out, the "soap" that is sold in stores isn't really soap. It is a detergent. Look closely and you will find beauty bars and moisturizing bars. Companies can't refer to their products as soap unless it is ACTUALLY natural soap. Natural soap is the result of a chemical reaction between water, lye (sodium hydroxide), fats and oils. This process (saponification) creates soap and glycerin. Glycerin is excellent for your skin! Glycerin attracts moisture to your skin and leaves your skin soft and moisturized! Did you know that commercial "soaps" remove the glycerin from the final product? They take it out and put it in things like lotion – that you will surely have to buy since your skin will be so dry and squeaky clean from using their "soap."

One thing I love most about making my own soaps is that I know EXACTLY what is going in to it. I choose the fats, oils, and everything else. And I know what they are! Here is a list of ingredients of a "beauty bar" that you would find at a store:

Sodium tallowate, sodium cocoyl isethionate, sodium cocoate, sodium laurel sulfate, water, sodium isethionate, stearic acid, coconut fatty acid, fragrance, titanium dioxide, sodium chloride, disodium phosphate, tetrasodium EDTA, trisodium etidronate, BHT, FD&C blue no. 1, D&C red no. 33.

I won't go on and on about how these chemicals are not good for our bodies. You know that. For me, my rule is if I know what the ingredient is and it is a natural ingredient, I will use it. Above, water looks like the only natural ingredient. Now you can see why these store bought "soaps" are called detergents. Protect your skin by avoiding toxic chemicals and use soothing natural ingredients instead!

Making your own soap saves you money!

What does a package of soap (6 bars?) cost you at the store? $1 per bar? Probably more, actually. I can buy my oils and fats in bulk. The last batch of soap made 12 bars. I should actually do a cost break down, but I am certain that I spend less than $1 per bar of soap.

Put your Essential Oils to good use!

Essential Oils are a great way to add a fragrance to your soaps! I can taylor each batch of soap to the current needs of our family. Since soap has a very long and stable shelf life, we can use them again as our needs change. For example, I may put lavender in a soap to help alleviate allergy symptoms and promote a calming feeling. The calming is great for my boys since they take their showers at night right now before bed. I might choose to use peppermint and lemon for a great pick me up to use in the morning! The options are endless!

Fragrances used in commercial products are incredibly toxic and can cause a host of issues! Most of the chemicals present in fragrances are known to cause cancer, birth defects, allergic reactions, and central nervous system damage. I do not want that stuff on my body, in my nose, or on my kids. Yuck.

It's fun!

Seriously, making my own soap – while totally intimidating at first – has been a chore that I look forward to! The process of it all totally fascinates me and I love trying new recipes!

Soap making safety guidelines

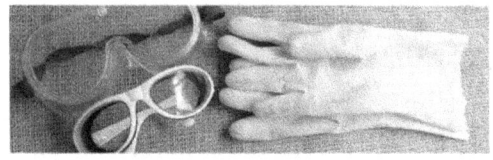

Safety is always first. Working with Lye and inducing a chemical reaction entails taking caution when attempting such procedures.

Research about your ingredients to understand what you are working with

Before you start, it is highly advised that you take your time to understand your ingredients. We will be explaining more about the ingredients in the coming chapters. For example, Lye is a substance to be treated with care. Spend some time getting to know about it for example, if you spill lye solution, don't attempt to neutralize it with vinegar. Instead, you need to rinse it with excess water.

Whether it splashed in your eyes or mouth or on your skin, rinsing it with water is the only and best solution to avoid skin or eye injury. If it spills on your clothes, remove the affected clothes immediately.

Follow your recipe

Chemical reactions need to occur in a certain way. It is all about proportions. Too much or too little of something can result in an undesirable effect. In soap making, all recipe ingredients are mentioned by weight, often ounces as you use traces of each ingredient. Therefore, it would be great if have your recipe printed-out so you can make sure of it, instead of fumbling with the phone or tablet while working with your ingredients, especially lye, you might risk spilling something. It may take you a couple of times to memorize the recipe by heart and then it would be much easier.

The second thing you need to follow your recipes precisely is a sensitive scale. Get a good quality kitchen scale or a digital scale. Make sure you test it out first with other known weights, such as a coin of known weight to confirm your balance's accuracy. Once tested, you need to weigh out all your ingredients as per your recipe. It is not advised to alter to change anything in the beginning. Some recipes mention percentages rather than weights which you can use to modify recipes according to your desired quantity but in the beginning, it is best to test with a prewritten recipe.

Take care of your eyes

Your eyes should be one of your number one safety priorities. A lot of things could go wrong and enter your eye during soap making, however, you can overcome this problem by wearing safety lab goggles. Lye or raw soap or dye powder all could find their way into your eyes, but not if you had safety goggles on. You should never skip this step. You also need close-by access to water to wash it just in case. If you want maximum visibility, consider anti-fog goggles.

Take care of your skin

Just like your eyes, the same is true for your skin. Lye or raw soap can be highly irritant to your skin if you were not wearing protective gloves. You can use latex gloves or rubber gloves. Dishwashing gloves are also fine but they can be bulky to work with. You could also protect your skin by wearing an apron or long sleeved top so that you don't have your skin exposed.

Ventilate your room

It is not advisable to work with a chemical reaction and the raw soap smell with closed windows. Keep the windows opened in the room that you are in to breathe fresh air.

Be prepared for spills

Even if you wear protective gear, anything could happen. That is why it is always important to have a plan B. Buy a granular absorbent or a universal absorbent spill kit and have this nearby. The spill could be oil, your soap, lye, etc. Always keep a water supply nearby.

Make sure you have printed the right recipe without any errors

Sometimes people can write anything on the Internet without having the appropriate knowledge of the percentages and calculations. Make sure you get recipes from trusted sources. You can use the recipes in this book.

Prepare all your ingredients beforehand

When you start, there isn't then time to go around your kitchen gathering or weighing the rest of your ingredients. Keep everything ready and within hands reach before you start.

Work with a clear space

Clutter is always a huge obstacle in any process. With lots of clutter, the chances of error increase. Always keep a clear working space.

Record your results and learn from your mistakes

It is important to record the results of your batches so that you can figure out what went wrong and avoid it in the future.

• Keep pets and children away

• Label the utensils you used for lye

• Be cautious but don't let that inhibit your creativity to decrease your fun

Chapter 11: Why You Should Toss Your Commercially-Produced Soaps

On an average day, people wash their hands an astounding 7-10 times! Though the blanket term of "soap" is applied to all sorts of things from the soaps used for dishes for the soaps used for cars, not all soap is composed of the same thing. The brightly colored soaps lining supermarket shelves have little in common with traditional soap. Though commercial soap has a bright and often delicious-smelling covering, these trappings are covering something quite different from the soap your grandmother used to use.

Commercially produced soaps both liquid and solid often contain artificial lathering agents, artificial colors, and countless unpronounceable chemicals—some of which can actually be quite harmful. For example, take triclosan, an antibacterial agent in many of the most popular soaps on the market. According to scientists, triclosan can increase bacterial and antibiotic resistance, cause skin irritation, and can even disrupt the metabolism. Other popular soap ingredients like pthalates and parabens can cause reproductive disorders and cancers.

It is tempting to drive to the store and buy soap. Commercial soaps are constantly marketed to keep consumers buying. Nevertheless, good marketing isn't always a good thing. Compare fast food companies marketing their unhealthy foods to commercial soap companies marketing their chemical-laden soaps. You know that these products aren't what are best for your body and that it's better to make them yourself!

The Wondrous Benefits of Making Your Own Soap!

Check the label on the soaps in your bathroom. How many of the ingredients can you comfortably identify? Triclosan, sodium laureth sulfate, methylparaben... The list goes on. Imagine what it would be like to know exactly what's in your soap by making it yourself!

Did you know that glycerin, which used to be an essential aspect of traditional soap, is separated out by commercial soap producers and resold to be included in more expensive beauty products? Natural handmade soap bars retain all of the good ingredients to moisturize your skin the natural way.

Creating your own soap, full of incredible essential oils and natural oils and fats to moisturize your skin, is not only fun but also good for your body. You will gain peace of mind knowing exactly what you're using on your skin. You can even gain more peace of mind from putting the right essential oils in your soap! Lavender, a classic soap ingredient, can relieve nervous tension, relieve pain, disinfect, and enhance blood circulation. Lavender's Latin name is Lavare, which means "to wash," no doubt due to its clean, fresh aroma. Blend lavender with other essential oils like cedarwood or pine to personalize your soap's scent and of course, its health benefits.

Not only is making your own soap good for you (not to mention an enjoyable hobby), but it is also extremely cost efficient. Making homemade soap takes more time than going to the store, but the results are certainly worth the extra effort. For most basic soaps, you simply need just four core ingredients: water, oil or fat, antioxidants, and lye, all of which can be easily acquired to make enough soap to give out as presents over the holidays!

Common Myths about Homemade Soap Making

1. It's too expensive.

Though the initial shopping trip for ingredients may be daunting, homemade soap is actually quite reasonable. One savvy soap maker calculated costs for basic unscented (and of course, homemade) soap at 15 cents per ounce of soap. Of course, purchasing ingredients in larger quantities will be more cost effective. Essential oils for fragrance can sometimes be pricy, so keep an eye out for deals online and in health food stores.

2. It's too difficult.

If you can measure ingredients, you can make soap! Making soap might have been very time consuming and difficult in your grandmother's time, but with today's modern tools, making soap can be about as simple as making a cake. A digital scale and immersion blender, though not essential for making soap, will definitely be an asset in your soap making process.

3. It's too dangerous.

Lye does seem like an intimidating ingredient, and you may have concerns over the need to use lye in your soap. As long as you are careful, there is nothing to fear. The lye reacts with oil in a process called saponification, and if you measure correctly, then there will be no lye in your final homemade soap. Just be sure to use glasses or goggles and kitchen rubber gloves to protect your eyes and skin from becoming irritated by the lye.

What Is Soap Making, Anyway?

Soap Making Overview

People have been making soap for thousands upon thousands of years. Ancient Romans are often credited with the discovery of soap, with the legend telling of fat dripping off an animal sacrifice, mixing with the ashes of the fire below it, and that mixture making its way to a river where women found their laundry much easier to clean with the substance. The hill the women were on was called Sapo, so the concoction was said to be named after the hill! Evidence has been found, however, of earlier soap making across the world.

Ingredients for soap making were commonly found from both animal and vegetable sources. Ancient Celts, for example, made their soap from animal fat and plant ashes, naming their product "saipo," from which our modern word soap may also be derived!

The first to produce soaps from vegetable oils and aromatic oils were Arabic chemists. These chemists produced perfumed and even colored soaps.

Soaps were primarily homemade or artisanal until approximately the eighteenth century. As medical science developed, the role of hygiene and the understanding of the relationship between cleanliness and health grew and popularized the concept of industrially produced bar soaps became readily available.

Commercial soap, as we know it today, came after the end of the First World War. Today, the soap industry is booming. What many people do not know about commercial soap is that similar methods of production are used today as were the 1800's!

The cold process method is most popular with modern soap makers, though some soap makers use the more historical hot process. Cold process soap is made from specific proportions of fats or oils and lye in a process called saponification, which occurs with very little heat. Soap produced by the cold process method takes approximately six weeks to be completely ready for use and can last for a long time.

Hot process soap, however, is a different take than the cold process method. In a contrast to cold process, hot process soap does not require as much scientific measuring. All the ingredients for the soap are put into a pot over a heat source and stirred continuously until all excess water has evaporated. The soap is then ready to use because of the higher temperature enabling quicker saponification!

Basic Soap Making Terms to Know

Acid
See "fatty acid"

Alkali
A compound with a pH greater than 7, also known as a base. Some examples include Sodium Hydroxide (lye) and Potassium Hydroxide.

Antioxidant
A substance that slows or prevents oxidation and helps prevent spoilage in soap.

Base

See "alkali."

Botanical

Related to plants or plant life.

Castile Soap

A soap made with a high percentage of olive oil, named for its origins in a region in Spain.

Caustic

Able to burn or corrode. Lye is also known as caustic soda.

Cold Process

A method of soap making that requires heat to melt oils but no direct cooking.

Cure

The time period between making the soap and using it. Cold process soap should be left for 4-6 weeks before its use to allow for the soap to completely saponify.

Detergent
A cleansing substance that acts similarly to soap, but is made from chemicals rather than fats and lye.

Emollient
Used to soften, smooth, and moisturize the skin, emollients are often vegetable oils and glycerin.

Essential Oil
A plant-based oil that has been harvested for its odor, flavor, or healthful benefits.

Exfoliant
An ingredient added to soap to help slough dead skin cells and dirt from the skin.

Fatty Acids
These compounds found in fats and oils give soap their lather, hardness, cleansing, and conditioning characteristics.

Fragrance Oil
Synthetic scented oil used instead of essential oil.

Gel Stage
A stage of soap making once it has been poured into the mold and becomes translucent.

Glycerin
A thick, sticky, and clear substance created during saponification, glycerin is also a natural emollient.

Hot Process
A method of soap making that requires external heat to cause quicker saponification.

Irritant
Substance that can cause inflammation or a painful reaction on the skin.

Lard
Fat that has been rendered from animals, often pigs.

Lye
Also known as Sodium Hydroxide, this is an essential ingredient in the soap making process.

Melting Point
The temperature at which oil for soap making melts.

pH
The measure of acidity or alkalinity of a solution. A substance with pH greater than 7.0 is a base, and less than 7.0 is an acid. 7.0 is neutral.

Preservative
A natural or manufactured chemical that is added to prevent spoilage.

Saponification
The chemical reaction between lye and a fat or oil to form soap.

Seize
Too quickly solidifying soap while still in the soap pan, seizing is caused by the soap

mixture having too much fat with high amounts of certain acids or some fragrance and essential oils.

Soap
The result of a chemical reaction between lye and fats or oils. If it's not made with lye, it's not soap!

Soda Ash
White powder that can form on top of curing soap.

Superfatted
The excess oils left unsaponified in finished soap that contribute to moisturizing qualities of the soap.

Tallow
The fatty tissue of animals.

Trace
The soap is ready at the trace stage, when soap spooned from the mixture and drizzled on top floats on top of the

solution for a short while before sinking back down.

Chapter 12: Soap Making Myths Debunked

Soap is a necessity for most people but few of them understand what it really is. Let's start by clearing the air on some common misconceptions about soap.

"Is soap really made of Lye? Isn't that stuff harsh on your skin?"

Here's the thing. Soap needs lye (sodium hydroxide) or another strong base like potassium hydroxide. It's basically composed of lye, water and fats. The Lye and the fat need each other in order to create a chemical reaction which allows the mixture to turn into soap and glycerin.

Water is just something to dilute the lye in. This reaction is called saponification. At this point, yes, the mixture is still pretty harsh until the lye has time to completely settle into the fat, but after a few weeks, the mixture should settle and what you'll have is soap with high glycerin content, much like the ones you see in grocery stores.

The harshness of soap all depends on its fat content. For example, laundry detergent soap normally has a 0% fat content because it's meant for things that are harder to clean. Soap for the skin is ideally needed for nourishment and moisturizing.

That's why body soap normally contains a 5-8% fat content. Any more fat added to the formula is a process called "super fatting" – like adding more moisturizing oils. This is the best way to make sure there are no more harmful lye molecules in the mixture.

In a way, lye is very harsh, but it is never intended to be used on the skin unless it's mixed with fat and saponified. In the end you'll have a skin friendly, non-harmful, glorious bar of soap.

"Is home-made soap really better for you? Some people say there's no big difference."

It's very different! Home-made soap far outweighs the benefits of other soap and you'll see that in the way your skin reacts to it. The smells, textures, and look of handmade soaps are not the same as the commercially-available stuff. Usually, the fragrance hits you right away even if it's non-scented soap. Its natural oils (walnut oil, avocado oil, coconut oil, etc) which come from fats are very unique in scent.

They usually vary in size as they are hand cut and are even heavier that store-bought soap because of their fat content. People who have sensitive, dry or itchy skin would love the chemical free moisture of home-made soap. When you use the soap you'll notice the bubbles are silkier in texture and afterwards you'll need less lotion.

Yes, there is a very positive difference in home-made soap and the results will be soft, supple and healthy skin!

"Some labels at stores say, 'Doesn't dry like soap.' Does soap normally make your skin dry?"

The things that make soap so good for your skin are the oils and fats. If the soap you're looking at in the store doesn't have these things it's likely to dry out your skin.

Beware and be extra careful when reading soap labels. If you see phrases like "cleansing bar," "beauty bar" and "deodorant bar", you better steer clear. These so called bars are not real soap and can often leave your skin cracked, dry and susceptible to germs and bacteria.

Not to mention they're more than likely chock full of chemicals and ingredients which are the leftovers from the manufacture of gasoline and motor oil - yikes! Among these chemicals are foaming agents and petrochemicals.

Petrochemicals sit on top of your skin, sort of like an extra layer. They are known to act as a barrier preventing your skin from protecting itself from toxins and wastes. This is why most store-bought soaps leave your skin feeling greasy or dried out. If you wouldn't put something in your body, would you put it on your body?

Chapter 13: Soap Making

Ingredients You Will Need

The following is a list of ingredients that you'll need to have on hand when you're ready to create a batch of soap. Again, it's better to have these on hand and a few different oils, so you have a choice.

LYE

Also called Sodium Hydroxide, it's an essential ingredient in both the hot and cold process soap making techniques. This caustic chemical induces saponification when it's mixed with a variety of fats and oils.

The Oils

Basically, when you're making soap using either the hot or cold processes, you're combining lye with an oil, like olive oil. Don't mistake these oils for of the essential ones we'll get about later on in the book. Essential oils are basically the essence of certain healing plants and herbs as well as provide an attractive scent to your product. When I first start soap making, I wasn't aware of the wide range of oils from which to choose to mix with the lye. And I certainly wasn't aware of the different advantages they brought to the final product. To give you a glimpse of what you can do even with your first batch of soap, I've included a short list of some of the common oils used in homemade soaps. Some of these I'm sure you've at least familiar with. Others you may never have heard of. In any case, once you know they exist, they open the door wider for a host of various soaps for your friends, family and even to help a soap making business, should you ever want to try your hand at that. I've also included a description of some of the benefits of using each oil.

Apricot Kernel Oil

With a shelf life of approximately six months to a year, apricot. This oil is a real skin pleaser. It's quickly absorbed into your skin. This makes it an excellent carrier for massage oil. It does produce small bubbles in your soap, so I try to keep this oil at 15 percent or less of the entire recipe. Most soap makers keep its usage down to approximately 10 percent. Shoot for that, especially on your first usage. Then you can always adjust the rate on later batches.

Avocado Oil

This oil makes a soft bar of soap. And is a popular one to use in the cold process method. Most soap makers have found that they have the best results with it when they use it at less than 20 percent of the entire recipe. Some even claim they've discovered that the optimal rate for avocado oils is 12.5 percent. There are several benefits to using this oil, not the least of which is the abundance of vitamins packed into it, including A, B, D and E. Avocado is a great addition to any massage oil if you ever decide to make them, as well as lotions and even skin butter. Not sure how long you can keep this oil and have it maintain its benefits? You can store this for about one year, after that you should purchase a new bottle, just to be on the safe side.

Avocado Butter

Not to be confused with avocado oil, the butter is solid as long as it's at room temperature. It makes the ideal ingredient for a wide variety of skin care products. In addition to soap, it's a great addition to balms and lotion blends as well as hair-care products. Avocado butter actually comes from the fruit of the avocado tree. It's then transformed into butter that is unimaginably soft. It has a nice, mild scent to it. When using it in your soap recipes, you'll probably want to keep it about 12.5

percent of the cold process method. I guarantee you'll love the result.

Beeswax

There are two types of beeswax: white and yellow. The shelf life for these is, well indefinite. You can keep them for years, and they should be just as effective as the day you bought them. What's up with the color difference? You'll discover that the yellow version is fully refined. The white variety, on the other hand, is naturally bleached. This occurs when it's exposed to thin layers of sunlight, air, and moisture. When you use it either in the cold or hot process method, it works as a natural hardening agent. You can use this at up to eight percent of the total of your entire recipe. You'll need to handle it a bit differently than the other "oils." You should melt it first and then add it to your soap when it reaches the thin trace stage. That's a minimum of 140 degrees. If you don't reach this temperature, the beeswax will just sit there hardened in your soap.

Canola Oil

Yes, this is the same canola oil you probably have right now on the kitchen shelf that you cook with. One of the biggest benefits of this oil is the cost. It's probably one of most inexpensive of all the oils we'll be talking about. That's something to take into consideration when you're just starting out, and you're not sure what to expect. When you do try it, you may want to consider using it with other oils, especially with coconut and palm oils. Doing this makes a 'balanced" bar of soap. Most soap makers keep the ratio of this close to 15 percent. Using this will give you soap that's whiter than if you used olive oil. That's a great attribute to keep in mind. That means you can use a wide range of colors in it. Talk about variety! Canola oil also releases a creamy lather that's often vital to a bar of soap.

You may want to consider substituting canola oil in a recipe that calls for olive oil at about 40 percent of your total oils.

Castor Oil

Of all the oils, this is probably one you didn't expect to see used in soap making. It took me by surprise, at least, when I first heard about. It's the same castor oil that so many moms through the ages have tried to get their children to swallow to help improve so many ailments. This oil will last up to a year in your kitchen without losing its effectiveness. Its thick and viscous nature comes from the castor bean plant. And yes, it does have a distinctive smell but rest assured, it's quite mild and not overpowering when worked into your soap. When you use castor oil in soap, it actually acts like a humectant. This means it takes moisture found into the air and puts in onto the skin. The other benefits of this oil is that it creates a wonderfully long-lasting leather. While some individual soap makers have made this oil nearly 25 percent of the total recipe, you may want to keep the ratio at approximately 10 percent. Most soap makers keep this ratio even lower at a range between 2 to 5 percent. I've personally found that using more than this only creates a soft and quite sticky bar of soap. Castor oil, though, is great for "superfatting." Because of this, it tends to create large bubbles in your soap.

Cocoa Butter

You've all no doubt heard how good cocoa butter is the skin. Here is your opportunity to use it to make your own custom soap containing cocoa. This butter will retain its effectiveness between a year to two years in your kitchen. At room temperature, it's hard, even brittle. That's why it's technically called butter and not oil. You'll find it's used in any number of beauty products. When you melt this though you should treat it in a manner similar to chocolate. It's best to temper it in order to avoid crystallization during the hot process method. If you're using it in the cold process technique, you don't have to worry about tempering it. Don't use cocoa butter at more than 15 percent of the entire recipe; even a smaller ratio works well. And keep in mind that the natural chocolate scent of cocoa butter may mask any gentle scents you may add to the bar.

Coconut Oil

This oil which seems to be gaining a larger devoted following day by day will retain its effectiveness even after a year of sitting on your kitchen shelf. It probably wouldn't surprise you to learn it's one of the most common of all oils used not only by the homemade soap makers but by the commercial manufactures as well. You can find the many types of coconut oil – some which can have varying melting points. The two you'll see most, though, are the two with the melting points of 76 and 92 degrees. This means it has one of the lowest melting points of nearly all the solid oils. Just as an aside, both of these melting points have identical saponification values. This means you can use both in the same recipe. An additional benefit to using coconut oil in a recipe is its outstanding reputation as a remarkable cleansing agent. It not only cleanses, but it produces large, delightful bubbles. The downside to this is sometimes it does its job too well and actually strips your skin of a part of its natural moisture. This leaves your skin dry. Some individuals have even experienced irritated skin. Most soap makers have discovered that a ratio of 25 percent creates the perfect balance without having to worry about drying out your skin. If you or the person you're creating this soap for has sensitive skin, then its best to keep this ratio to no more than 15 percent you can even useless if you want.

Coffee Butter

Here's another butter I had never heard of until I began soap making. It is a rich butter which makes it the perfect ingredient for any type of lotion, body butter, and yes, even soap. It's created out of a blend of hydrogenated vegetable oil and coffee seed oil. And, believe it or not, it really does contain some caffeine. The caffeine content ranges from half a percent to one percent. And in case you're wondering, it does have that natural coffee scent. Once you use your soap, you'll discover that the coffee butter contributes to a smooth and creamy texture to it. If you're using it in the cold process method, you don't want to use any greater amount than six percent ratio.

Emu Oil

Yes, you read that right. Emu oil. I wouldn't even mention it, but it's been touted for the last several years as a "miracle" ingredient that will cure, well, just about whatever is ailing you.

Supposedly it has anti-inflammatory as well an anti irritation properties. Whether that's true is debatable, but I've used it in soap with great success. It can be used in the cold process soapmaking method at a ratio of no more than 12.5 percent. You actually may want to use this oil at least once. It's said to be a 'skin-loving' ingredient. You may even want to combine this with essential oils that also have anti-inflammatory properties. Some of these essential oils include eucalyptus, anise and black pepper.

Evening Primrose Oil

This oil which is widely known has a reputation for effectively treating dry, or irritated skin. It comes by this honestly due to its abundance of fatty acid. It has a rather short shelf life in your kitchen, lasting only six to 12 months. If you decide to use it, you should use it at no more than six percent of your total oils in any cold process recipe. Now, you're ready to embrace and enjoy the more creative portions of the soapmaking process, adding the loving touches that make the soap uniquely yours. In the next chapter, you're going to learn about adding scents. At least you'll learn enough to pique your interest and discover even more when you're ready to continue your journey.

Soap Fragrance

Some people will choose to let their soap scent speak for itself and leave it to smell like simple, clean, handmade soap. Another idea is to use oils in your recipe like sesame or beeswax since they will impart their own unique and natural fragrances. I create an unscented soap fragranced only the natural aroma of oatmeal. It's proven popular with those with extremely sensitive skin. However, the most common way to scent soap is with either essential oils or cosmetic grade fragrance oils.

Essential Oils Vs Fragrance Oils

If you prefer the idea of natural scent then I'd suggest you'd stick with essential oils. They're concentrated plant and flower extracts and come in a fairly extensive range. The downside of using essential oils is their expense and propensity for fading with time. It's especially problematic for citrus essential oils such as lemon and orange. Fragrance oils are commercially produced perfumes for the toiletry industry. They're relatively inexpensive, have scent that lasts ages, and have a much more varied range to choose from. If you like baby powder scented soap or a shampoo that smells like coconut then you'll need to use fragrance oils. The thing I feel most uncomfortable about in regards to fragrance oils is that they are trademarked and patent protected. That means that you'll never truly know all the ingredients used to make them. In many cases fragrance oils are made of petrochemicals and allergens that cause people to sneeze or have skin reactions.

Scent Fixer

Above I mentioned that the scent of essential oils can fade over time but there are ways to 'fix' the scent so that they'll last longer. Sometimes another essential oil can help the others to stick and at other times it's best to use another additive that works to absorb the essential oils into it. Fixers are a bit more advanced in soap making but I thought I'd add them in so that those experimenting with making nice smelling soap aren't frustrated by their soap's scent evaporating during the curing process. Here are some of the choices you'll come across:

- Arrowroot

- Benzoin

- Cornstarch

- Oatmeal

- Orris Root Powder

- Essential oils

Soap Colors

In natural soap making you have several options for coloring your soap which will include powders you can purchase from specialty suppliers and even flowers and plants that could be growing in your garden right now. Your other option is to choose oils that will impart a natural hue to your soap. These could include clays, plant extracts, or ingredients that will caramelise and give a warm color to the finished product.

Oil Selection – some of your oils, such as olive oil, will impart a more yellow or creamy color. White and/or light colored oils will create white soap.

Clays – though limited in palette, cosmetic clays can add beautiful natural color to your soap. Clays can also create bars that lightly exfoliate and detox the skin.

Minerals & Micas – Mineral and Mica powders are available in a wide range of colors that can help you hit most of the hues of the rainbow. However, not everyone considers them natural. They're more accurately labelled as 'Nature identical' rather than 'Natural'. Minerals and micas are found in nature but are often tainted with unsafe heavy metals and are unsafe to use. That's why the ones available for mineral make-up and soap making are reproduced in a controlled environment.

Sugars – milk, sugar, and honey will caramelise if you add them to your batch before trace. They'll do the same thing if your soaping temperature is warm enough — over 105F in my experience.

Herbs, Flowers, & Roots – Nature creates all types of wonderful colors useful in soap making. Use calendula petals for golden orange, alkanet root for purples, and Madder root for pink. I even have a soap-maker friend who uses fresh Spinach to give her soap a brilliant green hue.

Chapter 14: Other Products To Make At Home

We have discovered that many people decided to create homemade soaps, both to save money and to make products that are truly green. However, is this always the best choice? Let's see the advantages and disadvantages of homemade soap.

Creating a soap at home is a way to save money and respect nature. The greatest benefits of homemade soap certainly exist in the abundant nutritional properties that can characterize the amalgam. Apart from the Fun Factor, those who love DIY and the ecology, find that the best thing to do is create bars of soap themselves, using ingredients that are as natural as possible! On the market, there are many types of soap, but these can cause allergies in people with sensitive skin: this is due to the chemicals they contain, including caustic soda.

We will decide, following the basic rules, which properties to give to our soaps: soothing, nourishing, toning. You can also choose which type of process should be chosen according to your needs: cold, warm, liquid, solid, semi-transparent, and whether it is to be used for body cleansing or for laundry.

The three ingredients used for what is called soap are: oils or fats, which are weak acids of animal or vegetable origin. The base oils or fats are those used in greater quantities in recipes, and they are also the least expensive and easiest to find. A basic fat widely used in Italy and Europe is olive oil, other conventional categories are sunflower, corn and soy peanut oils, while in the USA, palm oils or animal fats are preferred. Therefore, among the major advantages of self-production, there is the possibility of choosing the ingredients, the type of processing but above all, the savings. In fact, with a few ingredients, we can also obtain large quantities of soap that could be enjoyed for a long time.

The term nourishing oils refers instead to rarer, more valuable and more expensive oils that can give the soap itself a character or special properties. These include almond oil, jojoba oil, macadam oil, hazelnut oil, karate butter. Besides, the self-produced soap could also become an excellent hair shampoo. Being able to reach a production of this type is not very simple since we do not have the same tools present in the companies that allow you to obtain chemically functional hair products. With exercise, however, you will surely be able to obtain valid soaps that have the characteristics of shampoos.

Another advantage, not to be underestimated, is that you can choose the fragrance you prefer, opting for the addition of an indispensable oil within the compound.

4.1 Marseille soap

Marseille soap is a 100% natural product based on vegetable oils and sometimes essential oils useful for body care, face and hair thanks to the remarkable properties it has. Marseille soap is biodegradable and non-toxic. The quantity of caustic soda is calculated based on the "saponification coefficient" of the oil or fat used (olive oil = 0.134), while the quantity of water is approximately 30% of the weight of the oil.

As precaution, mouths, eyes and hands are protected by providing masks, goggles and gloves. Never use containers or tools made of aluminum, tin, copper, iron, cast iron, non-stick cookware and polystyrene. Choose stainless steel or heat resistant glass. Put the water in a container and just pour slowly while continuously stirring the caustic soda. The temperature could rise up to 100 degrees. Wait until it drops to 45 degrees, check regularly using a suitable thermometer. Simultaneously, heat the olive oil to 45 degrees. When both liquids have gone from the same temperature, pour water and soft drinks into the oil and mix quickly, with an immersion blender, while the mixture enters the "belt" phase. At this point, it will have become lighter and denser and by letting the mixture run from the blender, it will remain in relief on the surface. Here, the soap is poured into plastic recovery mold shaving lids, for easy extraction. Wrap in an old blanket for at least 24 hours. Once this phase is over, the solid soap can be removed from the molds. Following this, cut them into soap bars and leave them to mature in a dry and ventilated place for at least a month. It is preferable to handle it with gloves for the first two weeks.

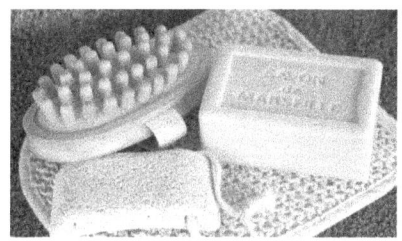

The soaps used on all days are not more than a chemical reaction produced by a strong base (usually sodium hydroxide)and a fat grass (long-chain carboxylic acid).

There are two different ways to make soap, the hot method and the cold method.

We recommend the hot method.

Every soap has a different effect on our skin, I will illustrate to you how the soap is made.

Let's see the necessary equipment and the ingredients to make them.

Equipment:

Electronic scales (the doses must be precise)

Some wooden spoons

Heat resistant pyrex containers

Stainless steel container

Oven thermometer

An immersion blender

Plastic containers or other molds, including wooden ones.

Ingredients:

280 gm of preferably distilled water

1 kg of extra-virgin olive oil

134 gm of caustic soda

4.2 Coconut oil soap

Soaps that have a high coconut oil content are very creamy and contain anti-bacterial and anti-fungal properties and soothes the skin without the use of harmful chemicals. The fatty acids help with the removal of dirt, dead skin and other skin impurities. Coconut oil soap is an excellent moisturizer for both the skin and the hair. The properties of the coconut oil also help remove dead skin cells. The oils also help prevent or reduce acne. They also help firm up your skin, and help you look younger as the soap is rich in antioxidants.

First, to make our soap we will keep having all the ingredients such as: coconut oil, olive oil, soda, coffee, coffee grounds, bran

Tools: Kitchen scales, stainless steel thermometer, gloves, protective goggles, mask, immersion blender, stainless steel pot, mixing bowls, stainless steel spoon, silicone spatula, stencil soap, baking paper, towel.

Settle into a well-ventilated area and wear protective clothing, goggles, mask and gloves. Pour 250 g of coconut oil and 350 g of olive oil into two different stainless steel pots. Prepare 225 g of liquid coffee in one bowl and 90 g of soda in another. In a third bowl pour 1 tablespoon of ground coffee and 1/3 cup of bran and then add the soda to the coffee and mix to dissolve. Warning: always add soda to the liquid, never the other way round. A chemical reaction will be started and the mixture will become quite hot, at this point put it aside. Now you can remove glasses and mask, not gloves.

Melt the coconut oil over low heat until the solid parts are removed. Add the olive oil. With a stainless steel thermometer, check the temperature of the oils and the temperature of the soda solution until both are between 40 and 50 degrees.

Pour the solution into the oils and use the blender to emulsify until the mixture begins to thicken and the consistency looks like a pudding. This process will take 5 to 10 minutes with a classic blender and up to an hour with an immersion blender. Once the soap has thickened, stir in the coffee grounds and oat bran with the stainless steel spoon or spatula.

Slowly pour the mixture into a soap mold. Lift and touch the mold against the tabletop a couple of times to release the air bubbles. Cover with baking paper, and then wrap the whole mold with a towel to insulate it.

After 24/48 hours, remove the towel and take the soap from the mold. Let the soap bar rest for another day to harden further before cutting into soap bars. Any sharp knife will work fine. A vegetable peeler can be used to smooth the sides if you prefer a perfect soap.

4.3 Vanilla soap

You can make vanilla soap only with a fragrance, as there is no vanilla essential oil. Although soap supply companies go to great lengths to make their synthetic fragrance sound like a true essential oil. Most people love the scent of vanilla, and often this scent is added to other scents, such as raspberry, sandalwood, lavender and orange.

The vanilla is famous for being a potent relaxer. Vanilla extract contains specific antioxidants that are vital in anti-aging skin benefits. These antioxidants can soothe wrinkles, heal damaged skin, and likely spice up an otherwise smelly anti-aging face mask.

Vanilla Soap revitalizes your skin cells and promotes its moisture retention capacity. As you bathe, the Vanilla Bean acts as a mild exfoliated while constantly releasing the fresh intoxicating aroma of Vanilla.

To make our soap vanilla homemade soap we suggest a classic recipe that combines creamy vanilla fragrance with hints of sugar and musk. Plus the addition of lanolin to this homemade cold process soap recipe makes this handmade soap not only feel extra luxurious in the bath, but it also makes it a great shaving soap by giving your razor that extra slip for a smooth shave.

You can "dress up" this vanilla homemade soap recipe with a touch of peppermint and a cream-colored layer in the middle by setting aside about a fourth to one-third of the soap after you've mixed the lye-water into the oils and it's reached a light trace but before you add the fragrance oil.

After setting aside a portion of unscented soap, add the vanilla fragrance oil to the soap in the pot and mix with your stick blender until you reach a medium trace. Pour half of this soap into your prepared mold.

Now add peppermint essential oil or fragrance oil to the soap you've set aside. If you reserved 1/3 of the soap add .35 oz. of peppermint essential oil or .9 oz. of peppermint fragrance oil. If you reserved 1/4 of the soap use .26 oz. of peppermint essential oil or .66 oz. of peppermint fragrance oil. Mix well with your stick blender to full trace then pour on top of the first layer of vanilla soap you poured.

Now pour the remaining vanilla soap into your soap mold on top of the previous two layers. Dust with pearl, silver, or white sparkle mica powder if desired then cover and set aside for 24 hours before unmolding and cutting your soaps.

Chapter 15: Best Homemade Soap Recipes

1. Cinnamon Soap

*Cold process

The cinnamon scent always reminds me of Christmas. Whenever I want to feel the magic of winter, I make this soap. The cinnamon scent will make your shower routine cozy, while also boosting your circulation. Coconut oil will feed your skin, and Shea butter will ensure softness.

You need 35% olive oil, 15% lard, 25% coconut oil, 15% shea butter, and 10% castor oil. Per 500 g oils: 1 tbsp white kaolin clay, 1 tbsp ground cinnamon, and 30 g cinnamon essential oil.

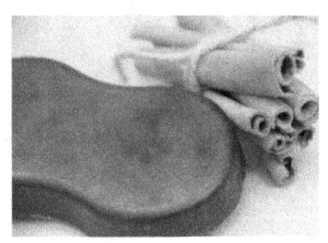

2. Green and Pure

*Cold process

If you are looking for more of an exploratory shower experience, this soap will do the trick. The combination of Patchouli, Spearmint, and Eucalyptus guarantee a powerful and rejuvenating scent, leading you into the world of love and nature.

You need 40% olive oil, 10% shea butter, 25% coconut oil, 20% lard, and 5% castor oil. Per 500g oils: ½ tsp green chromium oxide, 1 tbsp Australian Olive Green clay, 10 g patchouli essential oil, 10 g eucalyptus essential oil, and 10 g spearmint essential oil. 5% super fat.

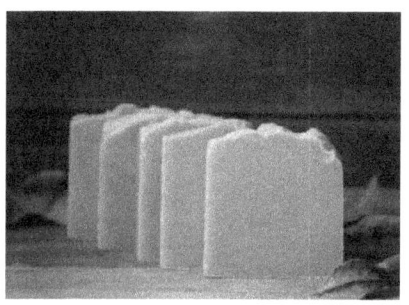

3. It is time for Gin & Tonic!

*Cold process

If you are a gin and tonic fan, then this is the perfect soap for enjoying these hot summer nights. This soap smells wonderful, and cleans your skin with ease.

You need 35% olive oil, 15% lard, 25% coconut oil, 15% shea butter, and 10% castor oil. Per 1.1 lbs oils: 26 g lemon essential oil, 1 tbsp white kaolin clay, 2 g juniper essential oil, and 2 Tsp orange dye.

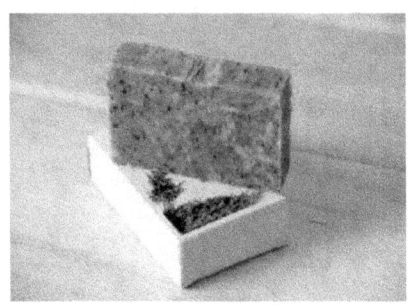

4. Castille soap

*Cold process

With commercial soap bars, you never know what is inside. So, the same goes for Castille soap that should be 100% olive oil. A true 100% olive oil soap will perfectly clean and hydrate your skin, while also being low suds. This means it doesn't create foam.

You need 100 oz. olive oil, 30 oz. Water and 12.6 oz. Lye.

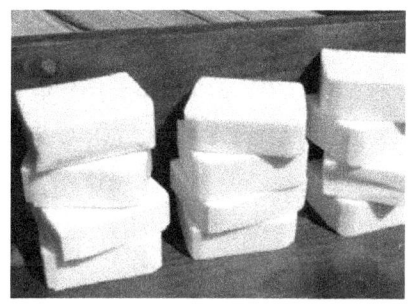

5. Take me somewhere far away from here

*Cold process

Rose scent is something we all love, especially on our skin. So, this Rose soap is ideal for bringing a romantic note to your nights.

First, you need to make rose petal infusion because, later on, you will use that mixture for the soap making process. In a jar, collect rose petals and set it aside for a few hours. After that, pour simmering water in the jar and cover it. Leave it for five to seven hours, until the water is pink, and then strain.

You need 28 ounces coconut oil, 12 ounces sunflower oil, 42 ounces olive oil, 11.73 ounces lye, and 26 ounces rose petal infusion. At trace, add 1 tbsp. of jojoba and rosehip oil, melted Shea butter, and two teaspoons rose essential oil.

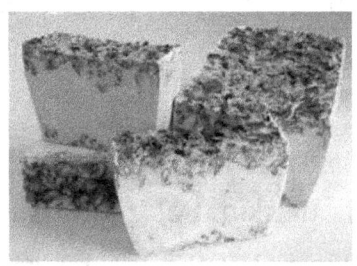

6. Bamboo Charcoal Soap

*Cold process

If you are looking for a rich soap that will clean your face deeply, this is the perfect recipe. Thanks to the oils and bamboo charcoal powder, this soap will give a refreshing and pure feel to your skin.

You need 30% palm oil, 25% coconut oil, 25% olive oil, 5% castor oil, 15% palm kernel oil, bamboo charcoal powder (1 tbsp for every 2 pounds of soap). For this recipe, you need a lye calculator, in order to determine the exact amount of lye, oils, and water you need. For making 2 pounds batch at 5% super fat, you need 8 oz olive oil, 9.6 oz palm oil, 4.8 oz palm kernel oil, 8 oz coconut oil, 1.6 oz castor oil, 12.1 oz water, 1 tbsp bamboo charcoal powder, and 4.7 oz lye (NaOH). If you want to make this soap smells unique, use lemongrass and peppermint scented oils.

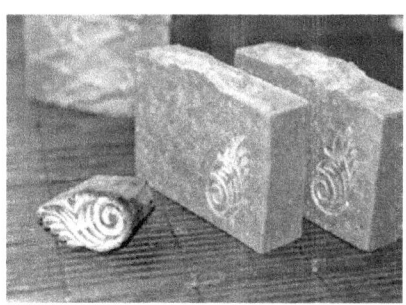

7. Calamine Lotion Soap

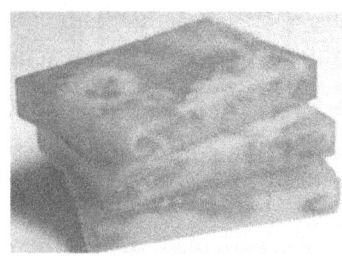

*Melt and pour process

In case you have a sensitive skin that irritates easily, despair not! For here it is your saver – Calamine lotion Soap. This is one of the most popular soap for sensitive skin, as it will soothe it, giving it just the right amount of moisture.

So, gather all the ingredients – 12 oz. goat's milk soap base, 5 Vitamin E capsules, 2 Tbsp. calamine lotion, 2 drops FDC Red #40 and ½ oz. bubblegum FO. Melt soap in a microwave or a double boiler, and stir in lotion. Then add color and Vitamin E. Lastly, add the bubble gum FO and your soap is ready to go into the molds. After it cools down, use a knife to cut it into bars.

8. Gorgeous and Delicious

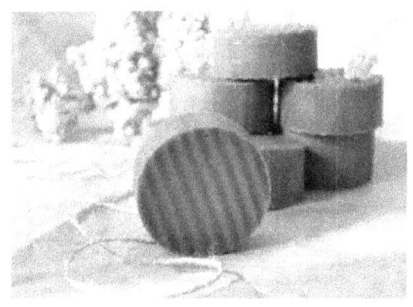

*Melt and Pour method

Who doesn't love chocolate? Well, I know I do. That is exactly why this recipe is one of my favorites. It smells so good and creates a real chocolate treat for your whole body thanks to its rich ingredients. You need 2 lb Soap Base, 1/2 cup Goat's Milk Powder, 1 tsp Macadamia Nut Oil, 1 tsp powdered Kola Nut, 1/2 tsp Cocoa

Butter, 1/2 Tsp Silk Amino Acids, 1/2 tsp Mango Butter and Chocolate Fragrance oil. After you melted the soap base, first add macadamia nut oil and silk and set aside to cool a bit. Then, add other ingredients.

9. Oldie but goodie

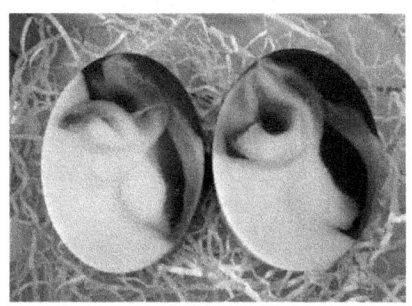

*Melt and Pour method

The well-known cocoa and vanilla combination is like a black cocktail dress – it can never be outdated. For those who can't resist this simple yet remarkably good mix, there is this recipe for cool-looking soap. First, you need to melt 2 oz. clear soap base and Cocoa powder in a double boiler. Then, set aside to cool a bit and add 10 drops chocolate fragrance. Pour into a mold, but only a half way. In another saucepan, melt 2 oz white soap base. You can add coconut oil and let the mixture cool slightly, before adding 10 drops vanilla fragrance.

10. The key

*Melt and Pour method

This luscious soap recipe is ideal for dry skin since it contains finely ground oatmeal for a gentle body scrub. Shea butter and cocoa butter will give your skin moisture it needs so as to look healthy and rejuvenated, while essential oils make this soap smell special.

You need 8 oz. shea or cocoa butter soap base, 1 Tbsp. cocoa butter, 2 Tbsp. shea butter, 2 Tablespoons finely ground oatmeal, 1 Tbsp. rose petal powder, 40 drops rose geranium essential oil, 20 drops ylang-ylang essential oil and 20 drops red colorant.

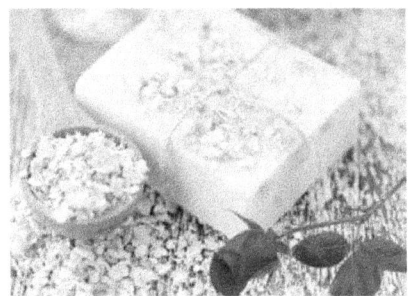

Conclusion

The next step for you will be to try new recipes than what has been provided in the book. You come up with new recipes or alter the recipes provided here to suit your needs. Do more research on the various soap recipes that are there, they are a plethora of them in the internet and guide books as well for advanced soap makers.

This will be a great way to spend your free time. With this as a guide, you can involve others to help you make soap like your children, family, and friends as a way to bond with one another and make it as much fun as you can, but with precautions. Or, you can teach others, if they have been interested in learning how to make soap.

Push your boundaries and start your own business by selling your home-made soaps and introduce new products like lip balms to your stock. This can be a great way to earn extra cash and it does not require you to work from 9 to 5.

www.ingramcontent.com/pod-product-compliance
Lightning Source LLC
Chambersburg PA
CBHW071844080526
44589CB00012B/1106